THE SCIENTISTS

WO$_3$ + 3H$_2$ → W + 3H$_2$O

2Ca(OH)$_2$ + ... → 2CaCO$_3$↓ + 2H$_2$

2J$^-$ → J$_2$ + 2

H-CE → HCE + (O)

Br$_2$ + 2e$^-$ →

Fe$_2$O

2 ROH

THE SCIENTISTS

a family romance

MARCO ROTH

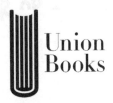

Union
Books

First published in Great Britain in 2013 by
Union Books
an imprint of Aurum Press Limited
7 Greenland Street
London NW1 0ND
union-books.co.uk

First published in the United States by Farrar, Straus and Giroux LLC,
18 West 18th Street, New York NY 10011 USA. All rights reserved.
Distributed in Canada by D&M Publishers, Inc.

Designed by Jonathan D. Lippincott.

A catalogue record for this book is available from the British Library.

ISBN 978-1-90-852619-9

1 3 5 7 9 10 8 6 4 2

2013 2015 2017 2018 2016 2014

For Imogen
and in memory of
Eugene Roth (1939–1993)

THE SCIENTISTS

OVERTURE

As usual, I'm beginning too late. My independent research report for biology is due in a week and I haven't even considered a topic. Somewhere between washing my hands for dinner, a foiled attempt to avoid looking at the bathroom mirror, and the walk down the hallway to the kitchen, I manage to suppress the sense that the situation is incurable. Perhaps, like the Romanov dynasty with their hereditary hemophilia, my family carries a recessive procrastination gene, held at bay for three generations of steadily ascending American life, until, in me, it burst into full expressive flower. This thought quickly gives way to the wish that my pubescent skin might somehow become spotless if I only washed my face an additional twice a day, a resolution I intend to carry out immediately. I return obediently to the bathroom, calling out to my parents to start eating without me.

At the table, where they haven't started, I begin, instead, to explain my assignment, my predicament. Excuses mount as my mother quickly dishes pasta onto my plate. It's not my fault I'm late. I'm busy, really. And am I really going to become a doctor, a scientist? I just spent two hours before dinner practicing scales, arpeggios, and the second violin parts for the youth orchestra (one hour, I admit, was actually spent slyly watching television or staring out the window at Central Park in anticipation of a scolding that never arrived). I attend the Friday meetings of the school's literary magazine club. I'm in the school play. Twice a week, I visit a psychiatrist, a few blocks from my school, as my father once visited a psychiatrist. Although he hates them now—they're not really doctors—he still pays for me to go, an unavoidable initiation ritual into a culture that believes no one should suffer, least of all in public.

Anyway, who can decide, at sixteen, who one is or what one should be? Isn't that the whole point of this "liberal arts" education I'm getting, to learn as much as possible about the world before becoming a person in that world? Plus, it's not even a real paper, like the ones my father used to write before his illness, "The Something Something of *P. falciparum*," the sort of thing that requires actual medical research. Just a glorified book report, a digest of existing discoveries, a test of how well we can summarize. I know how to summarize. I can write summaries of my summaries, that's how good I am.

My father dissects a piece of veal schnitzel he will eat less than half of. He complains that some microorganism has colonized his tongue, making everything taste like wood pulp or mush. I'd gladly finish it for him, if I hadn't recently declared myself vegetarian. Maybe I should write something like "When Good Bacteria Go Bad," or "Biology as Biography."

"You could write about reverse transcriptase inhibitors," my father says. And, before I'm even aware of having agreed, he takes control, staggering up from the table on unsteady, atrophied legs, returning a few minutes later carrying a heavy metal briefcase in both hands, already open. He sets it down on a pile of magazines at the far end of the table and roots around before coming up with several of the most recent articles on the things, xeroxed from scientific journals. He hands them to me and tells me to read them that night and ask him questions in the morning, when, he says, he's usually at his best. My father has given me the papers about the drugs that could save his life.

.

The next morning is not what my father calls "a good morning." I visit him in bed before I go to school. He may be feeling unusually weak, or feverish, or nauseated. I don't get into specifics. Over the last two years, there have been fewer and fewer good mornings, but my mother and I always ask him whether it might be one, as if repeating the question could influence the answer.

All the same, he makes an effort to quiz me about the articles. I understand well enough, now, that reverse transcriptase, although it sounds vaguely like some kind of learning disability, is the name of the enzyme that makes the AIDS virus so destructive of the human immune cells it occupies. A reverse transcriptase inhibitor tries to block that enzyme from working. The drugs my father takes, with their mysterious triple initials, AZT and DDI, actually are proteins—azidothymidine and dideoxyinosine—that somehow are supposed to trick a crucial HIV enzyme into bonding with them instead of the DNA components of the human immune cells the virus occupies, the way certain carnivorous plants are able to mimic the mating chemicals of the insects they feed on. The principle sounds simple enough, but I have no idea how this works, on the molecular level.

Like most sixteen-year-olds, I'm getting my science through metaphors. An enzyme, my biology teacher tells us, is like an ignition key that needs to fit a lock to start the motor running, or start any kind of process; every key, every lock is different. At the time, this is enough for me; I am not the kid in my class who is going to ask how such keys are made, or whether we can pick the lock. Keys and locks are the business of locksmiths or thieves. At Dalton, a private school on Manhattan's Upper East Side, no one plans on becoming a locksmith, while the thieves among us have their eyes on their parents' liquor cabinets or stock portfolios. Key into lock, so we can drive: the relation is what matters, not the mechanics, or so I think.

Instead, I imagine a gang of supersubtle saboteurs so lithe and practiced they will never set off an alarm. This gang, the HIV faction, for reasons of its own, breaks into a factory that makes parts for airport scanners. The gang members wield a special device that unlocks and reprograms the factory computers. This device is the reverse transcriptase enzyme. They then reprogram the assembly line, so that out of the same parts used to make airport scanners will come the very materials that allow the gang to slip, with all its equipment, undetected, from airport to airport and factory to factory. Once a factory is sabotaged like this, there's no possible way for it to go back to making what it's supposed to make. After enough of the wrong parts are made, the factory simply stops working at all.

Now I consider the factory owners. How do they stop this? They can change the security at the factory gates, but they don't yet understand how the saboteurs get in. They could try to check all of their employees to make sure none of them belong to this mysterious anarchist league, but it would take too much time. Instead, they try to sabotage the saboteurs, putting a special lock on their computers that will detect the device and render it harmless. So, the reverse transcriptase inhibitor. The only problem is that this new invention is unpredictable, secret even from the employees. Mistyping a basic password is enough to send the whole factory into lockdown mode, while perfectly innocent workers become suspects and are led away. No wonder my father can't get out of bed with all this action going on beneath his skin, or perhaps it's the effort to imagine it all that keeps him pinned there.

My father also understands—as I cannot—the process of reverse transcription itself, the way it really is, not just a metaphor. As he begins to describe it, he sits up in bed, jolted into action. A thin, mole-spotted arm, veins all too visible beneath the pale papery skin, reaches for a pen and legal-sized notepad from a drawer on the white dressing table at his right hand. The HIV virus, he explains, sketching a diagram of a cell nucleus, does something scientists once believed impossible. In a normal human immune cell, or in almost every other cell in the natural world, "DNA makes RNA makes proteins." That's the formula we copied into our notebooks. The virus, however, does the opposite. My father's diagram shows how HIV uses the reverse transcriptase enzyme, a protein, to produce a DNA copy of itself from its RNA. This is reverse transcription: a revolution in the microbiological processes of reproduction. The virus then uses another enzyme to integrate its DNA into the host cell's DNA, corrupting it. The immune cell's DNA begins to make more viral RNA, viral children, instead of the RNA that it needs to survive and function. It excites him, the deviousness of this virus, its audacity. He is a man who appreciates his enemy and wants me to appreciate it, too.

By the time he finishes his explanation, I'm late for school, the school I cannot wait to get to so I can get away from the other school my father has set up in his bedroom. Already I'm riding down four floors in the elevator, across the marbled lobby, smiling and waving at the morning doorman. Already, I'm boarding the M10 bus uptown and then racing across the middle of the street to catch the crosstown transfer, plunging, already, in imagination, into the crowds of the young, the healthy; people almost like me. I will keep my eyes down on my way to the back for a better look at the legs of the Dominican and Puerto Rican girls in Catholic school uniforms. Trying not to be completely obvious about it, I'll lean into the crowd, hopeful of a surreptitious brush with a pair of recently flourishing breasts. Early spring leaf buds wave in the branches along Central Park West.

I skip biology to play hacky-sack with our school's crew of misfits on the sidewalks of Eighty-ninth Street. Later, shouldering my way through the crowded fourth-floor corridor, I run into the teacher. His ponytail, checked shirt, though tucked in, and fondness for calling students "dude" mislead me into thinking he might be on my side in my one-boy crusade against the tyranny of deadlines and class schedules. Hedged in by a row of green lockers, I raise two fingers in an awkward peace sign. I was supposed to give him my topic today, did I have one? "Reverse transcriptase inhibitors," I tell him, and watch as he furrows his forehead as though wondering whether I've made them up. "You know," I say with well-practiced condescension, "how AIDS drugs work." His warning not to cut any more classes feels like an afterthought.

Riding this small triumph, I work through the week. The report's introduction proves an immediate obstacle. As much as I might want to, I must not mention that my father has the disease. It's been a secret ever since I started high school. I can't explain that he was the source of the articles I am using, that I hadn't spent weekends visiting the medical library at nearby Mount Sinai Hospital. I am, in a certain way, cheating, but cheating with good cause. Is it my fault that my home is a laboratory, my father both guinea pig and researcher? In any case, there are plenty of other reasons to be interested in AIDS in 1991. "The AIDS virus currently threatens humanity like no disease since the medieval bubonic plague," I write, in my best imitation of *New York Times* editorial-page bombast. "In New York City, alone, it is the leading cause of death among both men and women between 25 and 44 . . . For all the improvements of modern medicine, doctors were, until quite recently, powerless when faced with this mysterious disease . . ."

I want to go on to suggest that there is hope, that modern medicine has once again proved itself capable of saving the day, just as, in Eastern Europe, in the winter of 1989, those benign modern values of freedom and democracy triumphed inevitably over communism, that malignant mutation of freedom and democracy. Everything must connect, everything must be redeemable. But the hopeful conclusion does not flow so easily. Humans have their own reverse transcriptase enzymes, and the drugs are not yet finely tuned enough to distinguish between these and the virus's. Flooding a human body with reverse transcriptase inhibitors turns out to mess with all kinds of cellular reproduction: skin cells, immune cells, blood cells, neurons. Our bodies are always synthesizing proteins from RNA, and it's risky to interfere with any part of the process. A dissident group of scientists even claims that the symptoms we most closely associate with AIDS—wasting, falling immune cell counts and blood cell counts—are actually caused by these early-stage reverse transcriptase inhibitors.

Our family knows these side effects firsthand. The articles I'm reporting on are, in some cases, about drug trials in which my father participates. War is our textbook's favorite metaphor for the workings of the immune system and the various drugs we take to help it. We fight infections, eliminate foreign agents, go for "targeted strikes," but, as my father likes to say, faking a German accent, "Ve aim for ze shtars, but sometimes ve hitz London." Early retroviral therapy is a bit like this, like "killing the village in order to save it."

Making this even more complicated, "reverse transcription" is not a clean process. Errors occur, proteins switch places and shift shapes. Sometimes the mutant virus dies, other times it recombines to greater, more deadly effect. The HIV virus changes all the time and might be several different viruses. The inhibitor that works today may no longer work in several weeks, but it will continue to disable the same stable human proteins it always has.

I start to wonder if the drugs my father takes religiously, never varying from the prescribed regimen, are actually making him worse. Would there be more "good mornings" in a shorter life, less weakness, fewer indeterminate pains, if he stopped? Or will he be one more village destroyed in the name of Progress, the insurgents having already moved on?

Except I don't wonder these things, exactly, but, startled up from my desk, begin to shoot baskets on a small nerf hoop above my closet door, beneath the twelve-foot ceiling. I'm waiting for something, an idea, maybe. Perhaps I'm simply trying not to think at all, to avoid a certain mental arithmetic I plotted once: my father has had "full-blown AIDS" for two years, since I was fourteen, or a little before that; he told me only shortly after my fourteenth birthday. At the time, he gave himself between two and six years to live, although anything could happen. The drugs were progressing, but the exact match had yet to be found. I was now in my third year of high school. If I managed to spend all my time studying protein synthesis and immunobiology and everything else, even if I was some sort of teen genius—who was not, with one part of his mind, focusing on shooting free throws like the Knicks' point guard Mark Jackson, or wondering with another part whether the weather would be warm enough tomorrow for the girl who sat across from him in French class to wear a short skirt—I could not, even by superhuman application, hope to be a doctor and a scientist in less than three years.

I begin to feel less cheater than cheated. Is there a reason to study this if my father cannot be saved? If I will not be one to save him? What good is this kind of knowledge? With intense relief, I remember that there are still several chapters of *Moby-Dick* to read for English. Reading novels seems like the one uncomplicated thing I can do at this point. My parents don't think it's a waste of time, unlike sports, or going out on weekends, or acting. Unlike with music or math or science, I'm not frustrated by my inability to achieve instant perfection at it. Reading seems more natural and spontaneous than anything else I've been able to do for a long time.

And so, in mere moments, stomach down, asprawl on the bed, I go from would-be savior to nobody, "Call me Ishmael," not Israel. Down the hall, my father will be listening to something cheerful, maybe a Haydn symphony; he complains he can no longer listen to anything composed after Mozart. If he feels well enough, he might be sitting up in bed working on his translation of stories by Dino Buzzati, an Italian modernist author and doctor, or making his way through a favorite scene in Proust. I hear the quick pad of my mother's feet as she comes upstairs, and I wait for her knock, four soft taps. Her round face, hidden and framed by reddish curls and tortoiseshell glasses, flickers in the doorway, but she sees I'm reading and turns away, calling out a quick good night.

The next morning, wearing my unofficial uniform of black jeans, white T-shirt bearing a Japanese print, and my father's navy blue cashmere overcoat—he's become too thin for it—I trace a path across Central Park, a route I've followed for years. First I pass a couple of homeless men, camped out around a garbage-can fire in a small clearing behind the bushes at the Sixty-ninth Street entrance, then the morning's few joggers on the inner loop, those undeterred by stories of rapes and muggings in the wilds of the Ramble or along the paths leading to the reservoir. I walk due east, first, ignoring the dealers around the bandshell mumbling "Toke, toke" or "Smoke, smoke" into the collars of their army fatigue jackets—they don't have the drugs I want. On the other side of the park, I pass the sailboat lake, where my mother used to take me for ice cream on warm September afternoons when she picked me up from my first school. From there, nostalgic already for so early in the morning, I veer north, circling the Alice in Wonderland statue, then along the bottom of the sledding hill, and finally out to the embassy buildings and white stone town-houses along Seventy-seventh Street and Fifth Avenue. I duck into a more modest and modern brown brick building, off Madison, ride the elevator up eleven floors, and step into the burble of a white-noise machine and my unconscious mental life.

I understand I'm there because my father is dying, that I need someone to talk to about this who is not my father or my mother; that this white-haired, wooly-haired man, with his cashmere vest and framed diploma from Harvard, is the man I conjured up, somehow, when I went down to the kitchen one night, took the dishes out of the cupboard, where I'd earlier helped stack them, and began smashing them on the floor.

He sits stiffly, my psychiatrist, leaning forward, knee over knee, one wool trouser leg riding up to show he still wears old-fashioned silk socks with actual garters attached to a belt around the calf. I start to tell him about reverse transcriptase, and ask him if he thinks I should go to medical school. I'm not sure what I'm saying, exactly. He's my shrink, he's supposed to make sense of this mess, somehow. I don't know how much, but I know my parents pay him to take my scattered thoughts and tell me what they mean. Whatever it is, I've piqued him. From his leather armchair he lobs a question: "Are you so sure you want your father to be saved?" I pick at the laces of my Doc Marten boots. It will take too much time for me to undo them so I can hurl them at him, right before I take off my clothes and dance around the office naked. I know denial is powerless here. I understand I'm supposed to want my father dead, if not to kill him myself, unconsciously. My father has even been preparing me for it since I was around eight years old and he was beating me at chess: "You will hate me just as I hated my father," he used to say, sometimes after I told him I loved him. Admittedly, I haven't said that to him in a while. The inevitability of the man's question gives it a kind of unreality, as everything in the muffled plushness of my shrink's office feels unreal, as though I'm repeating a script rehearsed for generations. What do you say when confronted with someone who's certain you feel the things you do not feel and wants you to admit you feel them?

Instead, I tell my shrink that, while reading *Moby-Dick* last night, I came to realize my father is a bit like Captain Ahab, stalking the White Whale of the disease that gnaws at him. He is leading our family on a doomed voyage on which I'm just a deckhand, a sub-submate. But I also understand that Ahab is supposed to be all of us, at least all of America or Western Civilization or something. That we are locked in a death struggle with nature that we will always lose. I tell him I've often thought about not going to college but going instead to live in some kind of self-sustaining community somewhere like Vermont or outside Seattle. Suddenly, this idea seems absolutely right; there is no other logical or rational alternative than to give up the mad pursuit of mastery. My shrink half listens, then breaks in, "You're iridescing," he says.

I don't understand.

"It's like you're blowing these perfect little soap bubbles. Pretty thoughts. Elegant thoughts. But you're not thinking about my question." I say nothing and watch the final minutes of our fifty-minute hour click past on the clock my shrink keeps next to his notebook.

A week late, I turn in my report, one page torn and hastily taped where I ripped it in my impatience to detach the perforated printer-feed scroll from the dot-matrix pages. It seems to me a shoddy and temporary piece of work, an impression my A grade (marked down to A– for lateness) will do little to change. I sit with my father on a white couch as he feeds AZT, DDI, and a dose of antibiotic, antifungal, and antiviral medicines in through the IV that has taken up permanent residence in our dining room. My mother is usually the attending nurse, shuttling back and forth from the kitchen, bringing him juice or water, a piece of Entenmann's coffee cake—one of the only foods my father continues to find palatable. Its white frosting, he says, tastes of library paste, but not bad library paste. She also sets out *The New York Times*, or scientific journals. Between us is a silence, like the silence in the shrink's office, riddled with the question I must keep myself from asking, not because I want it but because I want it over with: "When are you going to die?"

·

These moments live again now as I write them. Twenty years on, they are present to me, although scrawled over by years, lives past and lives ongoing. They unfurl themselves, not just as they were, but spliced with other moments, like one of those medieval manuscripts recopied by generations of monks. Seeing myself then, I cannot escape the wish to scribble in the margin of my own consciousness that I was, as people say, a "wuss," that I failed to save my father. But that judgment is also the voice of me then, my sixteen-year-old self, who still wants nothing so much as to become a kind of hero. I want to make an unbroken storyline stretching from the child who once read tales of the experiments of Pasteur, Koch, Fleming, and other determined "microbe hunters" on the couch with his father—the same couch where that father took those potently inexact drugs I was powerless to change—to the man who would somehow make it right. That wish is also a romanticization, I can see. What I learned and what I failed to learn interests me, because, whatever I am, I am not an unbroken storyline. If I have a more-than-ordinary need to relive the past on the page, it may be because I have a more-than-ordinary fear of reliving that past elsewhere. My decision to go back through it all, as much as I can remember, was made to remind myself that I can consciously choose to make memoir out of memory.

1

The couch where my father died was also the couch where he taught me to read. I might as well start there: my alphas and his omega joined by a piece of furniture. It was a white sofa bed, pushed up against a wall the color of late summer nights. The room was supposed to be the apartment's dining room, but served more as my father's library. Sitting on the couch you faced two twelve-foot-tall bookcases, crammed to the top, with a third just like them on the right. The books both beckoned and frightened. Some of them were forbidden, placed high up on the top tier, after my mother once caught me leafing through a three-volume German history of the Second World War and its trove of Nazi photographs: glorious flamethrowers, the parade of tanks, the piles of corpses like so many broken dolls. Other books I didn't want to see at all. The cover of something called *Freddy's Book* showed a horned, hairy, and goat-footed man, hanging in a thicket of thorns.

"'Tis the eye of childhood that fears the painted devil," my father quoted at me, when I asked him to move it or turn the spine around. So the book stayed there, an object of dread, to admonish and terrify me until I grew brave enough to take it and read. It turned out to be a fairy tale about a misshapen but very human monster, a sort of Frankenstein's creature, who learned, in the somewhat happy end, to live with his deformities.

It wasn't a completely comfortable couch. The raised stitches on the cushion covers and armrests made it look hand-knit, but they left lines on bare flesh. I used to pick at the knots of fabric whenever bored or anxious during our weekend lessons. "Don't destroy it," my father said. English came first. The primer of choice, or at least the one I remember first actually being able to read, was called *Nobody Listens to Andrew*. The illustrations were Dick-and-Jane-like, a crew-cut boy in knickerbockers, girls in frocks with bows and neatly parted hair. The story, however, was not. Because nobody did listen to Andrew. He was just a boy with a busy family, a father who read the newspaper and smoked a pipe, older siblings, and in the end, maybe, Andrew ran away for an afternoon, or hid out in the treehouse in the backyard, or perhaps there was a bear lurking and he tried to warn everyone, but no one listened, turning it into an inverted version of the boy who cried wolf, a parable for a more responsive generation of parents. I never knew where my father found the book or why he'd picked it out. It didn't make much sense to me. I was an only child and everyone seemed to be listening to me all the time.

These first lessons were followed quickly by French, the seventeenth-century fabulist La Fontaine, "La Cigale ayant chanté tout l'été," we read together. Then I'd recite the tale of the ant and the grasshopper back at him, four lines at a time. That was classical education: "Repetition is the mother of memory," my father quoted again, as I stumbled over the lines at first. I kept up, eager to please, waiting to catch him in a secret smile of approval. Repetition may have been the mother, but my memory had a very visible father. Sometimes I was attentive, other times, leaning back, I'd run an imaginary rat through the maze of interconnected honeycomb moldings on the ceiling. Staring down, I'd idly trace the arabesques of the Persian rug with my toe.

When my wandering attention finally convinced him no further progress was possible, my father released me to entertain myself. I skipped off across the dining room along the carpet's red

rhomboid medallions, making myself go back to the beginning
if I missed a step, then jumped from peacock to antelope along the
hallway's animal carpet until I reached the open arch leading
to the enormous rectangle my parents called "the living room,"
although we really used it as a music room. It was barely fur-
nished: a small seating area with a couch and glass coffee table
at one end and the piano and stereo system at the other. The far
wall was a bank of six windows looking out onto Central Park.

Weekend afternoons, two or three times a year, the room filled
with a group of Chinese, Chileans, Poles, Italians, the random
Yugoslav, and Jews from New York's five boroughs, my father's
favored colleagues from the hematology and epidemiology divi-
sions of various New York hospitals. I was put in charge of opening our front door to the arriving guests, who included elderly
couples with Middle European accents from around the neighborhood, the shaggy poet who lived in the apartment across the
hall, my mother's musician friends. They sat on the rented chairs
I'd sometimes help unfold and listen to a string quartet run
through the program they would play at Lincoln Center the following week, or a recital of a Schubert song cycle, or, once, a brass
quintet my father had discovered busking outside in the park.
Their trumpets shook the windows and left our ears ringing.

I looked for my mother's curls bobbing up behind the pianist's shoulder as she turned pages, then I searched the rows,
trying to catch a cue as to how the music was going by reading
the faces around me. If someone met my stare, I'd shyly switch
to where my father sat on the edge of a black armchair, trying to
meet his eyes, gray behind his oversized black-framed glasses. He
hunched forward, his chin cupped in his palm during particularly complicated passages, the lines on his broad forehead creas-
ing, his broad lips pulsing gently, as if he were keeping himself
from humming along. He was overweight in those days, a pudge
of stomach visible when I caught sight of him in profile as he
greeted guests, his upper arms rolled with what I now recognize

as fat instead of muscle. I no doubt thought of him as bigger than he actually was. Although a couple of inches shorter than his father's six feet two, when he stood up at the end of the concert to thank the musicians and invite everyone for hors d'oeuvres he seemed, for that moment, to command the room. The rare moment when he stood next to my mother at the end of the evening, in the entrance foyer, as they saw our guests to the door, he seemed even taller. The top of her head barely reached his shoulder.

When no one was around, the living room was a lost continent, an America I could enter only by swimming across an expanse of open parquet until I'd reached a small kilim at the center. In quieter moods, I would lie on one of the rugs reading D'Aulaire's books of Greek and Norse myths or, absurdly—as it seems now— the Signet Classics editions of Shakespeare's history plays my father gave me after he'd taken me to see Laurence Olivier's *Henry V* at the old Thalia movie theater on Ninety-fifth Street. The seats at the Thalia sloped upward, the front row higher than the back row, in a way that forced your eyes to the top of the screen. I remember the battle scenes, the knights hoisted onto their horses by cranes, the whooshing flights of English arrows, and not much else. I cannot now tell what possible good it did me to lie there, warmed by the sun streaming over the trees, reading Shakespeare uncomprehendingly, making sure to ignore the notes. I lingered over the mysterious list called "Dramatis Personae." When I got further, I read mostly for the plot. I had perverse rooting interests, an odd sympathy for the murderous Richard III. Iambic pentameters did not come flowing out of my mouth. I was about eight or nine.

I'd lie on the carpet underneath my mother's Steinway B. It was a warm place. If my mother came in to play a Scarlatti sonata, for instance, or the accompaniment for a Schubert song, I'd listen while feeling the vibrations of chords and the thump of pedals push through me. Cadences and phrases flowed and mingled somehow with the patterns of the carpets. My father had

brought most of them back from Iran and Lebanon when he'd
traveled there in the early 1960s, but I ignored their provenance.
They were as eternal to me as meadows, and they were my meadows. Peacefully, I'd continue to draw out, in the weavings, what I
was sure must be the music I couldn't yet read, according to some
secret law of association now beyond recall.

My father wandered through and sat on a sofa at the opposite end of the room underneath a giant oak-framed mirror that
doubled the space. I'd watch him and my mother's reflection as
she managed her small hands and petite frame around the key-
board's widest intervals with only the rarest flaw. "She plays
beautifully, your mother," he'd say to me, rarely complimenting
her directly. This way of mediating kindness through me confirmed my sense that I was the center of our family life. Of course
he could simply have been performing an object lesson in kindness, telling me how much my mother needed to be praised. She
did need to be praised and she did play beautifully, although no
longer professionally, and then no longer even semiprofession-
ally, and then, gradually, hardly at all.

Who was to say if all this was good or bad? I was the definition of "precocious," which probably pleased my parents, but
nobody feels precocious at that age. The mixed shame and pride
of standing out only comes later. When I learned to recite "The
Crow and the Fox," in French, or repeated a joke in a Yiddish
accent to family guests, or sat straight, with my hands folded at
concerts, in imitation of the grown-ups I observed around me, it
was because I could do these things, make a game out of them. I
also knew my father would be ashamed of me if I didn't do them.
I grew used to an imperfect understanding, a shadow of meaning that fell across the pages as I turned them, incomprehensible
directions, a sense of an always wider world simultaneously close
to my grasp and beyond it.

I hid myself in the front hall closet, closed my eyes, and
pushed against the coats, going deeper, reenacting the beginning

of *The Lion, the Witch and the Wardrobe*, waiting for the moment when the hangers became tree branches and my mother's inherited furs became talking versions of the creatures they once were, live to the touch. I discovered I could give myself the illusion of a greater distance than was there by closing my eyes and reaching out into the darkness, expecting to brush the wall and thrilled when I didn't.

Other gaps frightened me: between the "train and the platform," as the subway conductors announced, also between the elevator and the landing. Our building's was an old elevator and didn't always stop perfectly, leaving a step up or step down and a glimpse into the shaft's void. I dreamed often of a world between the floors. Riding alone, I'd be let out somewhere that was like our hallway but not our hallway, the walls a darker shade. The people inside were not my parents. They were like them but older, and they kept cats, which we didn't, because they made the apartment smell like pee. "I live on the fourth floor," I'd say. "But where's that?" they'd say. Oh, I must be on the other side of the building, I thought. My mother was always talking about people on the "other side"—the building was in fact divided into North and South sides, joined by the common back stairway and landings where we left our garbage for the maintenance staff to carry down in the freight elevator they sometimes let me operate—so I guessed this was what she meant. The strangers would then let me out onto the back stairs, which turned into a narrow crawl space, the light growing dimmer behind me as I pushed on in the dark.

My mother remembers my childhood as a happy time. We were each of us alone together without rivalry or loneliness, restlessness or fear. The apartment was our temple: like the old Penn Station and the Metropolitan Museum of Art, but scaled down for domestic life. The architects had balanced openness and views over the park with cloistered spaces like my parents' upstairs bedroom and the kitchen, once reserved for servants, where the three of us clustered to eat at one end of a thick-grained table meant to seat eight. Under the high ceilings, even the heaviest pieces of mahogany furniture had only a friendly solidity to them, as if planted rather than placed.

My parents bought the apartment at the 88 Central Park West co-op in 1969 for $135,000. The Upper West Side then was an up-and-coming neighborhood, still considered edgy and derelict in places. Lincoln Center had recently been completed. Along Sixty-ninth street, musicians and teachers in cheap brownstone tenement apartments shared stoops with working-class Irish and Puerto Ricans who'd moved on up from Hell's Kitchen. The doormen lived a couple of blocks away, as did the cabdrivers; their parked, off-duty hacks punctuated the drab side streets with cheerful yellows. We met their children in a playground made of concrete-and-wood copies of ancient structures: a ziggurat boasting a slide, a Greek amphitheater for a sprinkler, a sandbox contained within the concentric rings of a Saxon hill fort. For the first few years, my parents' fellow co-op board members included a painter, a well-known poet and professor, a theater actress, a few doctors and lawyers, and several elderly and well-off Jewish refugees who had managed to escape Europe in the 1930s.

Maybe it was the early bourgeois bohemian character of the building or the fact that my father then earned only a modest researcher's salary at the Bronx public hospital where he also taught medical students, and had spent a fair amount of the money he'd inherited on his mother's death to buy the apartment—or simply that he'd grown up on the then-fashionable East Side, on Park Avenue—"The most boring street in the world," he called it— but, for some reason, he insisted we were "middle class." This phrase echoed through my childhood. It explained why we did not own a country house in the Berkshires or the Hamptons, like my friends' parents. It explained why my parents voted Democrat, why my father drove four-door Japanese compact cars, and why, instead of shopping for his suits at Saks or having them custom-made, he bought them, ill-fitting as they were, at Syms. It explained many things and also nothing at all, although it crucially shaped my sense of social justice. If "middle class" meant large apartments on Central Park West, then there was no reason why such housing shouldn't be available to most of us, in a truly egalitarian society. It was only logical.

For my father, the phrase invoked an acceptance of one's limitations as much as anything else. We were, according to him, a family of average height, average means, average talents distributed evenly, and average ambition. He said this one day shortly after I brought home my first low math grade, when I was twelve. I thought I heard a false note in this determined paean to mediocrity. Even earlier, I'd understood there were people my father called "Philistines": people who didn't listen to classical music, who watched sports on television, like my mother's father, people who were ignorant of world history like my father's sister, and who didn't care for art or literature like my mother's brother, an engineer; there were those who "preferred Coca-Cola to champagne," as my father wistfully said when Reagan beat Mondale (quoting Adlai Stevenson when he lost to Eisenhower). I'd seen actual, historical Philistines in my illustrated history of the Jews, "sea peoples," the book mysteriously called them, with beards, cruel faces, and spears, who worshipped fish-shaped gods like the one in my coloring book from the Metropolitan Museum of Art. I knew these people were the historical enemies of the Jews, that I was a Jew of some kind, though not the synagogue-going kind, or the Zionist kind, either; that although the Philistines outnumbered the Jews, the Jews still sometimes defeated them, as David defeated Goliath, and as Samson had, with the jawbone of the ass. It seemed then that my father meant me to be one of these Jewish heroes with unruly, curly hair like Samson's, to resist these invaders who'd brought him such grief.

Besides the Philistines, there were people my father denounced passionately as hypocrites. There were a lot of those: people who cared about school only for status or money; people who went to synagogue to show off their clothes, their daughters; people who talked about justice but wanted power or money or status, also called lawyers, like our distant cousin, Roy Cohn, the head lawyer for Joseph McCarthy's House Un-American Activities Committee in the 1950s. I knew a few other things about our family, things he'd begun to tell me—not directly, not exactly. They were legends, like the stories in the Bible, as remote from our lives as Abraham, Isaac, and Jacob.

There had been a poor man, once upon a time, Moses Philips, my great, great grandfather, selling bits of cloth from a pushcart on the Lower East Side. The poor man was a clever man, an industrious man, and his pushcart begat several pushcarts which begat a company that supplied material for shirts and so begat in its turn a company that made shirts my father never wore, Philips Van Heusen. The man had a son who took over the business. He moved from the Lower East Side to the upper reaches of Park Avenue, and that son sired a son of his own to take over the business, and also, as in a fairy tale, three daughters. The eldest married the heir to a paper company, the middle daughter married a banker, and the youngest married for love, a tall young lawyer, a sturdy swimmer and athlete born in the eastern reaches of the Austro-Hungarian Empire. Unfortunately, my grandfather was no hero or charming prince; he was a Grimm's-tale schemer, marrying for money. They had two children, my father the younger by four years.

He had been sent to private schools he didn't like and summer camps he hated. Boy Scouts were children dressed like fools led by fools dressed like children. A gentleman was a man with an expensive tie. A cousin of his was sent to military school for fighting a bully who'd been beating up my father. I'd learned that their world, both our world and not our world, the world he escaped from, was full of phonies, vulgarians, and frauds. Those people were not "middle class." My very name, European, ending in a vowel, my father once explained, was intended to be a symbolic break with those people who'd tried so hard to make my father "a real American." He'd been a junior to his father's senior, named after him while he was still alive, a deliberate affront to Jewish custom. This act of base assimilation, my father complained, robbed him of his identity before he'd even had one.

This, my father told me emphatically, was not to be my fate. According to my mother, he used to hold me aloft when I was a baby and say, "You are a person." He would say this to me later, too, although with various inflections. It was such an obvious statement, I was totally mystified by it. What else could I be? I was an only child of the "Free to Be You and Me" generation—despite my parents' distrust of popular music, we actually owned the record, the one where Mel Brooks is the voice of a baby girl who thinks she's a boy, William finally gets a doll, and fussy princesses get devoured by cannibals ("'Ladies first,' she said, and so she was, and mighty tasty too.").

"Free to Be" was an odd mantra for my childhood, especially because there were so many kinds of people my father obviously disapproved of. According to him, he'd basically given up on his own family when he was thirteen, reinventing himself as a changeling. He first did this through religion, plunging into his bar mitzvah studies. He'd briefly turned Orthodox and learned Yiddish, in 1952, well before the Yiddish revival movement became part of a more distant generation's nostalgia for lost roots. He spoke it largely to provoke his family, who had left behind both their language and sincere religious observance as remnants of the old country, reminders of the poverty and oppression they had escaped as though fleeing Egypt.

By rebelling through a resuscitation of history and discarded traditions, rather than by embracing the emerging counterculture of drugs and jazz—perhaps because this rebellion happened so early in his youth, before he had complete freedom of the New York streets—my father also, unintentionally, brought himself into conflict with what would become the dominant trends of American counterculture. The ordinary symbols of American rebelliousness were anathema to him. When the rhythms of the weekend drum circles in Central Park pulsed through our windows, my father declared it was "jungle music" for *"shvartsers,"* rock and roll was so much screaming or *"geschrei-*ing," even the avant-garde, contemporary classical music my mother began to take an interest in was only fraudulent noise.

As part of my middle-class childhood, my parents sent me to a half-French, half-English school, just across Central Park from us, on Sixty-second Street off Fifth Avenue. The Fleming School, despite its fancy location, was actually a daring experiment for its time and place, and middle class in exactly the way my father used the term. It was a small school—no more than two hundred children in kindergarten through eighth grade— overshadowed both by the Lycée Français, an official outpost of the French state educational system, and the richer and more pedigreed New York private primary schools, like the Ethical Culture School, where my father had been sent as a child. Ethical Culture had since moved within four blocks of our apartment, but he refused to send me, just as he refused to send me to Hebrew school, or summer sports camps, as had been done to him. I was going to be my own person.

2

I sometimes wonder how my parents' experiment in nineteenth-century, "middle-class" European education might have turned out if our family hadn't acquired a nonhuman member. Maybe the method's weaknesses would have become apparent sooner, revealed once I came into contact with Manhattan's ever-mutating cultural breeding grounds. My microscopic sibling, HIV, must have arrived sometime while I was in second or third grade, but I didn't hear about the creature until I was about to start high school. Exactly how I found out keeps melting back into a fog of memories: in one leadenly symbolic version, I'm interrupted while reading a letter from the girl I'd kissed a few weeks before. In another, I'm losing myself in a Yankees game, Mattingly batting in the bottom of the third—despite my father's best efforts to inoculate me against a sport played by "grown men in pajamas," as he called them, I'd contracted a love of the game from my mother's father, who'd been a teenage semipro player in the 1920s. My grandfather was already arthritic by the time he placed a bat in my hand, so I'd learned how to play mainly by watching the Yankees' first baseman, his deep crouch at the plate, weight on the back knee shifting quickly forward as he turned his hips to bring the bat through to meet the ball. My father is watching with me, for at least two minutes, a look of disgust on his face, like someone watching an alien mating ritual. He asks me to switch it off. I refuse, because I am a person, that is, until I notice his tone is pleading, not angry, and his face seems actually pained.

A third draft, written in graduate school while I was reading Diderot's account of a painting called *A Father's Curse*, tried a tableau of more unified family life—my father at his place at the kitchen table, opposite my mother, who holds a napkin to her face. The biology textbook he used when teaching medical students is placed to his right, open to the section on immunobiology. I've pulled around one of our high-backed cane dining chairs to see better, hunching uncomfortably over the edge of the table. As I press down into the wickerwork, a brief latticed tattoo etches itself on the back of my thighs. The tattoo looks like the diagrams of molecules on the page. My father, sitting straighter, stretches a finger over the book, pointing out a section or chart of the various kinds of cells that make up our immune system. I imagined the scene as one of a series of drawings: "My father explains the mechanism of the disease that's killing him."

In the latest version, my father tells it as a bedtime story, as if I were a small child. Maybe he's lying on his bed, exhausted, although it's only early evening, in his usual blue boxers and white undershirt. He calls out to me as if already at the last reserves of his strength. And I—years later, protesting still the changes that day would bring—switch us around into what seems a more natural arrangement of parent and child, my father standing over me as the summer twilight deepens over the park . . . "Once upon a time," my father says, in the tone he used to tell me stories of Semi Semmelweis and the Romanian Robbers or the amazing and true discovery of penicillin, "when you were about five or six years old, I was working on an idea I'd had for a new malaria drug. I was also supervising the sickle-cell clinic at Mount Sinai Hospital, and most of the blood we used for experiments was taken as samples from our sickle patients. One day, as I finished drawing blood from one of the regulars, I did something very stupid. I wasn't wearing latex gloves, which you're supposed to do whenever you're handling blood, and, as I was about to get the needle out of this guy's arm, he jerked and the needle came out suddenly and poked me in the wrist, just below a vein. It was in for no more than a second or two. Now this guy had a lot of problems, not just sickle-cell disease, but, like a lot of the patients, he'd got hooked on heroin to get rid of the pain. You remember that's when I came down with hepatitis; you were too little for me to tell you about it. But at the time we were beginning to hear about this new disease . . ."

I didn't really find out in any of these ways, although each of them approaches some kind of composite fragmented representation. Something happened, unmistakably, because before I went away to a music camp for the summer I knew nothing, and when I started high school I knew my father had contracted HIV at some point, now had full-blown AIDS, and, according to him, had anywhere from zero to five years to live. There was one more thing I knew, which had been impressed upon me: I mustn't tell anyone about it.

What I actually remember most vividly about my initiation into my father's secret life as a dying man was the sensation of air-conditioning. It was August, around my father's birthday, his forty-ninth. My father loved air-conditioning, as he loved veal scaloppine, breaded or in a marsala sauce, red wines, old historical films on TV (anything with Errol Flynn or about World War II), a good stereo system, a firm mattress. These were the few physical pleasures of his dying years.

He loved the white noise as much as the coolness. Only two things can really quiet New York City, snowfall in winter and the persistent hum of an air conditioner's motor in summer. The drum circles and bandshell concerts in Central Park faded; the blaring horns, sirens, and car alarms were turned into muted background accompaniments to an evening spent in front of his Marantz speakers. Later, I'd realize that he loved the machines for the same reasons he became a scientist and placed his faith in modern medicine. The AC, although we never called it that, brought comfort and showed us our capacity for benevolent domination of the earth. He took pride in it, the same way he'd tell me stories of how malaria had been eradicated in America and most of Italy by draining the swamps and killing off the mosquitoes with insecticides. These were concrete signs of progress, of hope for the world, like the Zionist project to make the desert bloom, or, at least, to install air-conditioning in Jerusalem and Tel Aviv.

My distrust of the sacred AC—later confirmed when I learned about CFCs, ozone holes, and global warming—probably began that same night, just before the start of high school, when I heard about my father's disease. I'd just survived six weeks without any aid from artificial coolants at a music camp in the middle of Tennessee, where the heat and humidity exceeded even New York's. They had been happy weeks and seem happier now for being the last of my childhood, or the first and last of a more promising adolescence. I'd loved wildly, promiscuously: first, the twenty-year-old violinist from Buenos Aires who sat next to me at breakfast the first day. She immediately adopted me as her young admirer, letting me tie back her long black hair before rehearsals, teaching me how to pronounce Spanish, Argentine-style: the double *ll* of *¿Como te llamas?* pronounced with a soft *sh* sound, with a hint of *j*. There was my neighbor in the boys' dorm, a Korean flutist who introduced me to the highly unclassical music of the Cure, which was also how, one night in his room, I met the girl whose letter I was reading sometime on or about the moment I learned my father was going to die.

She probably didn't fall for me so much as the stories I told her about the wonders of New York—the nightclubs I'd never been to and the museums and concerts I had. She was a girl of the Blue Ridge Mountains, the first self-consciously rebellious person I'd met, already dreaming of escaping her town. ("You must come visit," I told her, as I walked her to her room after our last orchestra concert, and she reached out her hand, her nails painted dark purple, and circled my wrist.)

Clearly, I could never speak to her again. Her impression of me was utterly false. I'd become another person. What sort of person, I wasn't yet sure. I grew cold in my room, still air-conditioned, and tried to make sense of my father's impending death. All men are mortal, my father is a man, my father is mortal. He was going to die sometime in my life. It would be sooner than we thought. To keep the secret, the important thing was to behave as though nothing were wrong. This was what he said he wanted. I would still do my homework as I had the previous winter while my father was hospitalized with "an allergic reaction to dust from the painters redoing our dining room," or so my mother told me when she suddenly packed me off to my aunt's house for a few days. He actually had *Pneumocystis carinii*, then one of the leading killers of AIDS patients. I'd known nothing about it. He could have died while I was writing an essay about *To Kill a Mockingbird* for Mr. Adams's eighth-grade English class.

My parents were even sending me to France for the last two weeks of summer before high school. "We want you to be your own person," they said, independent, uninfluenced, unafraid, possibly unconcerned. I'd spend a great deal of time picking at the paradox of such impossible imperatives: "Be free," "Enjoy yourself." Did they just want me to go away? Or were they strange hypocrites, saying what they thought was the right thing to say and hoping all the while that I would also say the right thing, which was that I didn't really want to go away at all? Or maybe, through desperation or delusion, they really meant it, they really thought I could grow up strong, happy, and, yes, oddly unburdened in spite of everything.

I went off on a tour of the Loire valley and Provence with the family of my closest friend from Fleming, an unruly kid with wild black hair and a monumental Roman nose. He'd played me my first Madonna song, showed me my first *Playboy* magazine,

taught me the word *pussy*. We used to play complicated war
games requiring battering rams and battle cries—"*La gloire ou la
mort!*"—eventually leading my father to bar him from our apartment. "The Geschreier," he named him.

From that trip only one scene remains: On a rocky outcrop-
ping above the Avignon bridge, that great stone fragment that
breaks off a third of the way across the Rhône, my friend and I
were talking about our first year of high school ahead. He had it
planned out: the yearbook committee, soccer practice. His older
sister's friends gave him advice on how to pick up girls, how not
to be a geek. I'd follow him a little while longer, as though he
had the secret of an easeful and successful life, but it was probably
then that I knew we couldn't stay close. I watched the river beat
against the ruined bridge, the bathers happily splashing their
tawny bodies farther down the bank, the fishermen absorbed in
their lines. According to his parents, I was a terrible guest, moping
and complaining as they drove around visiting châteaux, vine-
yards, and Cézanne's enormous white mountains. I found that out
when my father yelled at me later, saying I'd embarrassed him.
But I hadn't told them a thing.

Secrecy came easily, at first. It felt like the natural condition of
adolescence, along with its counterpart, gossip. They fed off each
other. We all had secrets: crushes, ambitions, jealousies, and sor-
rows, most of these still concealed from our everyday selves. I
would no sooner have blabbed about my father's illness than
I would have let my mother find the stains on my sheets. Our
housekeeper, one of my earliest crushes, had been let go, for reasons I couldn't quite understand, and my mother began to do
most of the washing, in addition to the cooking she'd always
done. She also spent more and more time in an earlier era's "maid's
room," off the kitchen, which she turned into an office. My father
called it "the junk room." There she began to train herself in the

ways of the nonprofit arts of grant writing, fund-raising, and career counseling.

Despite the ease of keeping quiet, I wasn't exactly sure why it was necessary. As I began to pay attention to the AIDS stories proliferating in the newspaper, I wanted my father to be brave. I wanted to tell him I was proud of him, not protect him. It was 1988, a period when the growing AIDS-awareness movement needed "innocent victims"—that false category—to show the disease was more than "God's punishment on drug addicts and homosexuals." Jerry Falwell or Pat Robertson or some such televangelist called it that, and my father liked repeating it ironically, in a mock Southern accent. Around us, my father was never quiet about humanitarian politics or his belief that biology was beyond good and evil. He took the Hippocratic oath seriously and applied it globally, as a form of ethics. Only a few years earlier, he'd joined a group of doctors and musicians protesting the use of torture by U.S.-supported regimes worldwide in their "dirty wars" against the left. He'd visited torture victims in Danish hospitals and signed petitions. But now, facing death, near certain but slow, he suddenly developed a terror of softer forms of persecution.

"I could lose my lab," I remember him saying to me once, perhaps when I'd asked him if I could tell my favorite English teacher. "Is that what you want? The hospital wouldn't want the publicity or the risk. You have no idea what people will say. Think about your mother: all her friends watching her suffer, calling up to see how we're doing, but really to make themselves feel better. They don't need to know." This made sense; humiliation was always a slip away. The Dalton School, for all its progressive principles, was not a place where one wanted to be noticed for the wrong reasons.

One of the biggest common secrets we carried around was how hard we worked. We were all in ferocious, sometimes friendly competition with one another, but over two competing kinds of status: grades and social standing. The "smarter" you were, publicly, the more people hated you and the more your social stock tumbled. The best way to deal with this was to pretend that you were doing no work at all, that the test didn't matter. The worst way was to become an authentic slacker instead of a faux slacker; then your grades went down and your social standing, while perhaps improving in the short term, did not mask the growing contempt of your peers or salve the mounting anxiety that you might have to go somewhere like Union, Trinity, or Oberlin instead of the Ivies for college.

For whatever reason, I was no good at this code. I failed at it before I learned to reject it. I didn't care about grades as such, but I did care about appearing clever. It was supposed to be the opposite: cleverness was shown by pretending you didn't care, and I never got that straight until it was too late. I was one of those kids you could always make cry or reduce to violent tantrums with well-placed cruelties. The Geschreier and I fell out pretty quickly once high school started. I'd noticed he was avoiding me, trying to get in with the lacrosse team kids. "I will not be your proverbial sacrificial lamb," I told him. He thought this was hilarious and for weeks I was "the proverbial sacrificial lamb." My father was right. It was dangerous to put oneself out there. And yet I did it again and again and do it now. The boy who was about to become my closest friend had a term for it: "being Jesus." "There you go," he'd say, "being Jesus." He said it because he thought it was true, and I agreed with him, although he couldn't hide his smile of satisfaction, the cruelty that comes when we're able to tell our friends unpleasant truths about themselves.

Oddly, until I was being persecuted (always unfairly, for something or other), I thought of myself as invisible. I looked around at everyone as though I'd never come down from the cliff above the Avignon bridge. My father's mortality stirred me with a strange kind of pride. I had my secret, the most important secret of all: we were going to die, the lacrosse captain, the violin prodigy, the math genius, the banker's daughter with the Matisse paintings on the wall of her Fifth Avenue apartment. Neither hard work, nor talent, nor money would protect them, and it was my privilege to know it.

That first year of my father's full-blown AIDS, our kitchen transformed into a medical school cafeteria and a sort of war room where we followed the course of the illness. Blown-up photographs of lesions wound up on the table, a few places down from where we ate spaghetti Bolognese. My father and I practically dared each other to eat while looking at electron microscope slides of nematodes, while my mother left the table in protest, her food untouched, and took refuge at the piano. We studied Kaposi's sarcoma or looked into the milky, worm-ridden eyes of people suffering from river blindness. These other pictures were there for perspective, as though we were telling ourselves how much worse it could be or was about to get. My father knew that if he'd been African he'd already be dead. But he couldn't really know what was going to happen to him and he couldn't really prepare us.

After such dinners, he'd climb the stairs slowly and retreat to his bedroom. Sometimes I remembered to clear the table before going to scratch out Mozart's fourth violin concerto, in A major. I was always embarrassed to replace my mother's perfectly turned phrases with my own halting notes, and even more embarrassed that she'd be listening. If she corrected me, I'd fly into a rage, and, in this way, destroyed two music stands, one fairly expensive bow, and three neck rests. My mother treated these eruptions like outbreaks of bad weather. She waited them out under some mysterious mental shelter until they passed. My father, upstairs, mostly ignored them. We were each of us alone together.

Of my father's disease, the most important thing, there were, as yet, few visible signs. He'd been losing weight, but he'd been trying to lose weight for years. People even complimented him on the success of his diet, he announced with grim satisfaction. The pneumocystis pneumonia left him with only the occasional cough, and his numerous allergies had all vanished.

The way my father explained it, the HIV virus, once it enters the bloodstream, seeks out a special kind of white blood cell to use as its host. The "helper" T cell, as it's called, usually triggers an immune response that allows us to make new antibodies or increase the production of those we already have. As the virus breeds over years, T cells decline faster than they can be made. Without these T cells to generate new antibodies, our immune system turns inefficient. Antigens, or "foreign agents," go unrecognized and unfought.

This slow stripping away of the barrier between what our textbooks called "self and other" is what makes AIDS a hideously creative condition. Misdiagnoses were normal. No one knew people could suffer from a common cat virus before they began to do so. Ordinary drugs might backfire extraordinarily. An antibiotic made from a fungus, used to kill off a bacterial infection, could run out of control, breed in your throat, or even affect the brain. A population of benign bacteria in our intestines that helps us digest food might grow suddenly wild, stealing nutrients we need to survive. If nothing else got you first, you might slowly starve to death.

My father tried turning his thoughts into a substitute immune system. Encounters with strangers, or even friends, animals, undercooked or odd foods, these were threats to be anticipated. He wouldn't walk around the street wearing a surgical mask, but he often had a handkerchief and seemed to move as quickly as possible from our apartment to his car to his lab, each an enclosed and relatively safe space.

My awareness of his need for constant mental discipline over his body made sense of a great deal of my earlier childhood: why he'd always turned aside my requests for pets, why he'd abruptly stopped our wrestling pillow fights when I was seven, and—by the time I was fourteen—had stopped touching me at all, why he disliked fish in any form, would eat cured ham but never shellfish, why the mention of any Third World country invoked a monologue on filth and disease and the perils of poor public sanitation, which he immediately made fun of himself for getting into. Quoting someone else, as usual, he'd usually end by saying that Americans like to confuse toilets with civilization.

He was also infectious, at least to some. Like any *New York Times*–reading child of the '80s, I knew that AIDS was a sexually transmitted disease. I also knew, somehow, about sex—at least I'd been forced to take our tenth-grade sex ed class. I was relieved to know my mother hadn't been infected, but that raised uncomfortable questions about my parents. What hadn't they been up to? My father said he'd known something might have been wrong since I was six. Perhaps the disease was the real reason I was an only child? True, my father used to insist that siblings were terrible and he'd never do me the disservice that had been "done to him," even though he was the younger brother. He used to prefer the French term *fils unique*, because it seemed more dignified than the restrictive and lonely "only child." But he also often—and with increasing frequency—told me he'd really wished for a girl, usually when I was doing something particularly boyish. His nieces, both older than I was, were held up as shining examples: quiet, studious, they set up a soup kitchen, they helped around the house. Girls were kinder, matured earlier, were more obedient, loved their fathers without competing with them, he explained. Rather than try to become a girl, I just began to tell myself that I'd needed a sister and now knew why I didn't have one.

Our apartment was large, the walls thick. I was often away from my parents, or they from me, during the summer or over vacations. I always had great difficulty thinking of them as sexual beings. Perhaps it was a kind of only-child possessiveness, in

which each parent existed only for me, never for each other, but
there was little enough to make me think I was wrong. My parents' bed, for instance, I always thought of as my father's bed; he
was usually in it, my mother usually not. It was a scene of in-
struction, a place to listen to music, for reading and rest.

At fourteen, I could not understand what might have attracted my parents to each other. I'd come to view them through
the all-judging eyes of adolescence, the young New Yorker's restless, relentless schooling in the ways of beauty. Every morning
I'd be greeted by the black-and-white torsos, breasts, hands, even
sometimes the faces of lingerie-clad models opposite the contents page, A2, of *The New York Times*. Coming home from
school, as I stooped to gather the mail, there in *The New Yorker*
and *New York* magazine, both of which my parents continued
to receive long after they stopped reading them, would be different models, this time in color, sipping drinks or lounging, dresses
billowing, from the balcony of some tropical hotel. I saw such
people on the streets, too, around school, emerging from taxis,
or at the opera. From the standpoint of fashion, my parents remained frozen in the '70s. They lacked the trimmed elegance of
their parents, or seemed to have rejected it. I found myself hoping that looks could skip generations, but my disgust at my parents was no greater than my growing disgust at my own reflection.

And yet, could it have been . . . Yes, my father really did give
me condoms! Before I left for Tennessee, where my violin teacher
had recommended I go study with a friend of hers. The shame
of it, the absurdity, at the time, how farcical it made actual sex
seem. How strained, too, that moment, as though he'd told me
to go fuck with his blessing and then attached the curse of pre-
caution, another self-consciousness added to my own. If I could
have explained it to him, I would have said I was more interested
in desire than its consummation, or that it would be enough to
be noticed. As it was, I could barely stammer thank you in the
embarrassment, the mystery of it all. I also couldn't help think-

ing that my father hadn't been paying close enough attention. Was his barely teenage son, slight dark fuzz already growing above his lips, really about to talk a girl into letting him put one of those things on?

We never forgive our parents for good intentions poorly put into practice. The sense of betrayal somehow feels more complete. But, even then, I thought I could divide intent from effect. There was a strange closeness in our relationship: my father and I discussing our bodies with detachment, or rather he lecturing and I learning to ask questions. T-cell counts, acne—anything was fair game as soon as I could get my tongue around a multi-syllable piece of mixed Greco-Latin medical jargon. On long car trips, when I was still practically a toddler, my father would say, "we'll be there faster than you can say *colojejunostomy*," or *adenosine triphosphate*, or *deoxyribonucleic acid*. Often, these trips were to visit my father's father, who I'd been told was dying from a prostate tumor the doctors had caught too late. "Why couldn't they take out people's prostates before there's any cancer?" I'd asked. I also begged to have my appendix removed once I discovered it was useless but potentially harmful. I was, at certain moments, capable of being the coldest rationalist. What was an organ, a finger, a leg, compared with the survival of the whole?

If my father wanted to make a doctor of me, which he never said he did, he'd at least succeeded in making me a believer in the power of scientific information. On occasional weekends, when I was in middle school, he took me along to his laboratory. He let me spin the blood samples in the centrifuge while he set up the microscope. Then he'd show me slides of blood cells and parasites; teach me how to recognize the infected cells, the cobalt-dyed twists of parasites lurking within the red blood cells they'd colonized. My father's voice guided my perceptions as I fiddled with the focus knob, and I always half wondered whether I was seeing what I was supposed to because it was there or because he wanted me to see it.

And how did my parents see their teenage son? Were they proud, ashamed, anxious? They told me they wanted me to be just like a normal teenager and I tried not to disappoint them in my ordinary gestures of rebelliousness. A DO NOT DISTURB sign appeared on my door. Led Zeppelin and Dylan, more often than Bach and Beethoven, played loud enough for my father to condemn "the herd of wild elephants" stampeding out of my boombox speakers. I spent hours on push-ups and sit-ups in front of the mirror, attempting to will myself into some alternate body that someone might look at with something less than revulsion. Photos of models made their way onto my walls. My favorite was one from *National Geographic* that showed only the head and neck of a headscarf-wearing Afghan girl whose improbable yellow-flecked, ultramarine eyes stared out, without reflecting, on a world of suffering I could scarcely comprehend. I'm in love with her and she's already dead. It's hopeless, I told myself. The photograph would become famous later, when we'd all become more familiar with that part of the world's cycle of pain and revenge. Back then, the photo was only part of my secret teenage pathography, as if I recognized in her some kind of dignity or stoicism I guessed I'd need, but which seemed to exist only in the Third World or ancient history books.

When I turned sixteen, my parents wanted me to take SAT tutoring classes. "You're hypocrites," I said in my father's voice. They wanted me to cheat using their money. If I was smart enough, I'd be okay. If not, I would take my proper place. They enrolled me in the classes, but I never went to them. I understood this was part of some process of becoming free, that freedom meant freedom from one's parents. I didn't understand why they wanted me at home at all to give them grief. With perfect irony, whenever my grades slipped or I was making too much noise, my father would say "off to military school with you." In good moods this was accompanied by or replaced with his humming *"Non più andrai, farfallone amoroso . . ."* from *The Marriage of*

Figaro. Other times he just said it with no particular inflection, and I wondered why he didn't just carry out the threat. I began to sleep the deep, unbestirrable sleep of the teenaged, burrowing into the covers against the eastern sunlight over the park. Some mornings I showed up at school at ten o'clock. "Are you on drugs?" my mother asked me, once or maybe twice. It was after that that I smashed the dishes and found myself a week or so later at my psychoanalyst's Madison Avenue office, by myself.

Why go after the dishes? That was the obvious question for my shrink to have asked, and the answer was not "because my father has AIDS and is dying," which is what I might have said had he asked it. Somehow, however, I knew I was there to talk about my dying father, not my behavior, which I always thought of as a reaction, as unpredictable and uncontrollable as volatile chemicals combining in a tube. My mother told me that her grandmother was rumored to have been a great smasher of glassware . . . as though this were built into our DNA, an unfortunate trait I'd inherited, but nothing we could control.

Going to the shrink made me happy, at first. It was the most normal-feeling thing I'd done for a while. Even hating my shrink felt blissfully natural. My friend, the one who liked accusing me of "being Jesus," had a shrink of his own. I had been jealous of his shrink, and now I didn't have to be. He told me his older sister had HIV. This was my soul mate. We were brothers together in our closeness to suffering. I'd told him about my father, finally, as we walked homeward one afternoon, down the most boring street in the world, where nothing was ever meant to happen except an endless parade of taxis. I spoke quickly, nervously, as if the doormen we passed were waiting to steal the secret from me. I thought my confession cemented our friendship, having made him both witness and accessory to my betrayal.

If I felt lighter, freer, happier for having a true secret sharer, not just a paid confidant, I could no longer face my parents without shame and anger boiling up at the slightest pretext. Secrecy falsified everything, even the telling of the secret. I'd sworn my friend to keep quiet, of course, and of course he had to tell at least his girlfriend, who told someone else who'd known me since kindergarten. And this person came to feel I looked down on him, otherwise why wouldn't I have told him first? By the time I graduated, it was possible that anyone who knew me and my friend knew about my father, which meant, in all likelihood, most of the school knew and kept it from me. This did not, for me, make the secret any less secret or less powerful, nor did it make me feel any better for having talked.

3

My guilt at that teenage betrayal comes back now, as I write this, not with the old savagery but stained with something often called maturity. What sort of injunction forbade me from speaking the truth to a kid whose confidence I hoped to earn? But *confidence* is a tricky word, charged with multiple meanings. If I'd showed more confidence in myself and my besieged family, perhaps I wouldn't have needed to exchange a confidence in return for more confidence. Maybe I wouldn't have demoted myself from the ranks of teen supermen in order to share in the ordinary human misery of shrinks, gossips, pity parties—"community," in short. I can still feel, however dimly, the shame of violating my parents' code, so why have I decided to do it again, as though, having told one or two, I might as well tell the world?

Familiar reticence might have taken hold of me again, if my father hadn't pronounced the punishment I was, with some irrational foreknowledge, always expecting. It seems almost funny now. It started when I determined to live out every privileged American child's rite of passage and send myself away to college at my parents' expense. "You have to get out of New York," my friend had said. My shrink agreed with him. I needed space. I had to stop worrying about my parents. My father was getting thinner day by day, but he said, not quite cheerfully, that he wouldn't die for a while.

I turned down my father's alma mater, Columbia University, for a chance to follow my friend out to the heavily manured pastures and Ultimate Frisbee fields of Oberlin, Ohio. When I announced my decision to my parents, they maintained the first principles of my upbringing—I was "my own person," "Free to Be." Besides, the approval of my analyst counted. Much as my father hated Freud, he never said he was wrong, only unscientific. When I'd packed my bags, my mother gave me a quotation from Petrarch, "It's not the place that ennobles you, but you who ennoble the place." My father sent me off with a sentence of his own, setting a trap I'd soon spring: "You'll be disappointed," he said, hiding what he must have felt behind switched pronouns and tenses.

I was disappointed. Over Oberlin's long winter recess, I went to Mexico to study Spanish and live with a family in Guadalajara. It's not that I didn't miss my parents, but I had no idea how to act with them, or with anyone else. It seemed simpler to do everything in another language, which was like acting anyway. I barely spoke to the other Oberlin kids on the program. Most of them were stoners who seemed to be following some script called "self-liberation" marked out by Kerouac and the Beats. I could almost sympathize with these kids, which is what they were to me, or envy them, although I had no wish to be counted among them. I, too, had picked up *On the Road*, thrilled by the sentences whizzing by at the careening speed with which Dean Moriarty drives from New York to Baja. I, too, could feel the open window, the boundlessness, the joyous wildness of sex, not for love but for self-celebration, or rather celebration of the human animal, so different from my parents' sense of personhood. It was seductive, but also false, hysterical. Perhaps I'd caught the note of elegy behind the ecstasy—"I even think of Old Dean Moriarty the father we never found, I think of Dean Moriarty, I think of Dean Moriarty"—as if the kind of life Kerouac thought to be best, the only life he actually believed worthy of that name, proved unsustainable from the beginning.

My loneliness in Guadalajara still comes over me sometimes. I've felt it while walking the in-between zones of New York, along the car shops and old warehouses of Atlantic Avenue, or happening by the coffin manufacturers just up from the Gowanus Canal. It's a liminal, lost sensation of having wandered wide, endless boulevards, among rows of orange trees, winter butterflies, seasons reversed and out of order, dogs barking from behind fences meant to keep out intruders. It's not the place that impoverishes me but I who bring my own sense of poverty, of loss, to the place. It's a sense of near nothingness, as though I were not so much a blank slate as an erased chalkboard, still bearing illegible smudges of smoothed-over writing.

This same feeling redoubled when I finally touched the Pacific Ocean after several hours of meandering bus rides over mountain roads. I'd gone as far away as I could while still being the person I was. Within me, still, there was a dying father, an anxious mother waiting in an apartment in Manhattan, and what they felt too and what I felt about them were still an unshakable part of capital-L Life, as were the books in my father's library, the concerts, the file folders filled with his medical records. It might have been a lesser life, but it wasn't the opposite of life, much as I sometimes felt it was. Perhaps I'd found my true self in Mexico after all. To go any farther and rid myself of these images of my parents, of my lost feeling, it seemed I'd have had to free myself of the whole white-man, Eurocentric mess, become—God knows—a simple fisherman in a hut, attuned only to the pulse of waves, seasons, blood spurting from the fish I'd gutted meeting blood from my finger where I'd cut it while gutting the fish—flowing blood without test tubes or centrifuges. When I got back to Ohio, in early February 1993, I called my parents and told them I was putting in a transfer application to Columbia.

I was accepted, in April; I imagined my father might have called in a favor or made a donation from some stashed family reserve fund I didn't know about. I never felt certain that college was earned, or that I deserved to be there. When I got the letter, I felt I'd let someone down, but couldn't say who. It occurred to me that I was disappointed only because I didn't want to disappoint my parents. Maybe that emptiness was part of what it really meant to become my own person. To return to New York suddenly seemed an act of cowardice, of surrender, equaled only by my having left the city in the first place. I filled out Columbia's acceptance form, but secretly kept myself enrolled at Oberlin. I guessed the first tuition payment for the fall semester wasn't due until later in the summer, and assumed I'd have a clearer sense of what I wanted by then. I was keeping my options open, something that seemed the special right of people like me. There was a place for me, the right place, a home that would make me happy if I'd let it.

I nurtured my secret "bipolar" alternative until the beginning of that summer, when an Oberlin tuition bill must have found its way to my father. And so I was summoned once more to our once-library, almost completely converted into my father's private hospital room, white curtains placed over the glazed French doors. I was glared down at by volumes of Heine, of Dante, of those history books in German and French and Italian, medical books dealing with the care and rehabilitation of torture victims and malaria and sickle-cell sufferers; rebuked by IV bags, rubber gloves, and needles.

My father spoke: I had no sense of what was good for me, he said; I'd always messed everything up through clumsiness or in-attention, or perhaps was evil, as when, at age four, summoning some demon of provocation, I'd called my babysitter the N-word in an attempt to drive her away and make my parents stay with me, which they did, causing my father to miss his aunt's seventieth-birthday party, and when I gave up on Hebrew lessons at age seven for the joys of baseball, or, when I was ten, while staying with his friends in the South of France, had managed to partially miss the toilet one night, stumbling to pee in the dark.

No minor transgression had gone unrecorded in his memory, and, over the years it seemed he'd spent biting his tongue, they'd grown from slips into symptomatic failings of my flawed character. I'd squandered the attention, not to mention the money, $200,000 and counting, that he'd lavished on my education, and only he, dying as he was, stood between me and the absolute ruin I was about to make of myself should I return to that hippie cow college, which he regretted ever letting me set eyes on.

My father's verdict came down instantly: I could return to Oberlin, if I wanted to, I was my own person after all, but, if I did, I would forfeit my inheritance. I would be on my own. Here was the punishment I'd been waiting for . . . And it caught me completely by surprise. I felt it was the grossest unfairness, a devastation of everything I had believed my family to be. Although I deserved to be punished for failing to keep my father's secret through high school, as he'd required, it made no sense to be attacked on this entirely different front, to be kicked so wildly into the cold. My father had always made references to Rousseau's "noble savage" and natural morality. I'd been taught to believe in the natural goodness he'd believed in, not original sin. Until that point, he'd almost always acted as if I'd vindicated his confidence; instead, it seemed, I'd failed at every moment when, unknown to me, he'd put it to the test.

His methods, it's true, were not always consistent. There was the time he'd thrown me to the ground and kicked me because I was playing a loud game of air tennis while a chamber music group rehearsed in our living room, and the curious way he had, whenever I made the mistake of mentioning that I was interested in any of the things I was beginning to be interested in, of reminding me how I'd once, when I was five, said I wanted to be a garbage man, "and even if you become a garbage man, I will still love you and your mother will still love you."

I thought I could take the kicks, but in a few spoken paragraphs, my father had not just threatened me but damned me. If I went back to Ohio, I'd be an ingrate who'd abandoned his dying father and soon-to-be-widowed mother. If I stayed in New York, I was a mercenary who honored my father only for the riches he'd bestow on me when he died. Money had previously played almost no part in my thoughts about anything, for it had been another part of my father's educational philosophy to keep me free from thinking about it. I'd never had a fixed allowance, never been encouraged to take a job. I could buy whatever I wanted as long as it was "reasonable," which meant as long as it was an expense my parents approved of, such as books, or a new computer. Nothing but conscience obligated me to think about where that money came from, whose additional sweat and blood let my parents buy the plane ticket to France, who decided that it was in my best interest to cut ten thousand jobs so the stock prices in my mutual fund would improve, to charge those high prices for drugs. I couldn't even be sure that I wanted my family's money at all.

There was only one honorable response to my father's threat. I had to stand up to the dying person he was in the name of the living person he'd once tried to be. If I couldn't save him or keep his secret, I could at least save certain ideals, ideals I'd recognized when I read Emerson's essay "Self-Reliance" in my last year of high school. If I was not meant to be a heroic scientist, I could at least be a nonconformist. Ignorant of the specific religious history of the term, I took the word to mean an antihero, an independent social exile: family, pedigree, class, these things would mean nothing to me. I would accept the status of the outlaw. We would soon be dead to each other anyway, no matter what happened. So I resolved to go back to Ohio and then even farther.

I plotted my emancipation, rode up midtown elevators to meet with our family accountant to see how much money my father—irrevocably—had set aside in my name when I was born. I phoned the Oberlin financial aid office and was sent a folder. I wondered whether I should hitchhike out to the Midwest immediately, or stay with friends in Manhattan while putting the forms together. Which friends would take me in, and how did one go about filling out such incomprehensible instructions? Should I say a separate goodbye to my mother? She had said nothing, done nothing, withdrawing to her small office off the kitchen as my father and I raged at each other.

"Tincture of Time," my father's prescription for almost all non-life-threatening ailments, makes this whole episode seem embarrassingly melodramatic now, like watching a black-and-white film reel of a Yiddish theater production of *King Lear*, all thick shadows and ghostly white makeup, much ripping of cloth and beards, a play performed in translation and in the wrong medium, and, so, difficult to recount and difficult to imagine anyone caring as much about as the actors themselves once did. As drama, it had all the lurid poignancy of true tastelessness.

To my knowledge, my father never changed his will. The whole thing was a private drama without any visible consequences, a kind of fit made worse by my inability to treat it as one. Whenever I told people about my father's "will shaking"— mostly they've been psychiatrists—they usually suggested, in a kind and pitying way, that he must have been "clinically" insane. It's true that he was very sick by that point. It's entirely possible that one of the legion of foreign microorganisms cavorting around his body could have got to his brain. Forms of dementia, say the doctors, are common in late-stage HIV sufferers, and toxoplasmosis—that cat disease—has been said to cause "personality change."

Impending death may also cause personality change, or it may bring out all the fears and uncertainties stored up over a lifetime, and harden them. Our family had gone through the looking glass: what we found there was no more time to tell ourselves that things might not work out so badly, no time to say the boy is still young, or that there are some virtues that need years to mature. All those everyday and often necessary lies lost their staying power. I could not tell if my father was testing me or capitulating. Either he was giving me up to the same forces that might have once ruined him, or I was being used as a last pawn in the endgame of a chess match he'd been playing his whole life: against his parents, against his class. I was either going to become a new queen, the most powerful piece on the board, or be sacrificed completely for the sake of a game whose rules I had not yet fully understood.

One solution was to learn to play a different game entirely, to make my own rules, become truly autonomous. But when it came to striking out on my own, a kind of inertia took hold. Going on felt as tedious as returning. When my father pronounced my disinheritance, I was already halfway to Columbia, living under a cousin's name, swiping my way into a dormitory suite on 114th Street and Broadway with her borrowed ID, taking "Structure and Style," a summer writing course at the School of General Studies. I'd even found a job clerking at the Shakespeare & Co. bookstore, then on West Eighty-first Street. A late July afternoon, coming out of our writing class, a girl walked beside me through Riverside Park. As afternoon became evening, she suggested we see Kurosawa's *Seven Samurai* at Symphony Space, next to the old Thalia. It turned out to be her birthday. Her boyfriend was away for the summer, working in Washington, while she'd stayed, she said, because of a campus job that was too good to pass up. I told her a bit about my needing to choose between one place and another without letting on much about why I needed to make the choice, or what it meant for me if I did. The next week, she put a note in the campus newspaper personals, "Marco, I hope I see you in the fall." It gave me some hope, but I couldn't

say what for. So I did nothing, or rather I surrendered condition-
ally. I would go to Columbia, as my father had demanded of me.
But I wouldn't have anything to do with him, I told him. I would
obey the letter of his law, like the Ivy League lawyer he now said
he wanted me to become.

4

One afternoon, shortly before the start of the Columbia semester, when it seemed I could still chuck everything and go west, I went to say goodbye to our family friend C. I'd loved her hopelessly, for a long time, with a more hopeful hopelessness than I loved my Afghan photograph, the infinite hope of a four-year-old who believes he will one day be grown up enough to marry his mother—or at least his older sister. She was the first one, the only one around me, who made me think life might be a good thing and not a dark joke. Thirty-two years old that summer, she'd come to New York out of the Midwest, in her twenties, with an English degree, a love of classical music and classical musicians, baseball, Brahms and Bill Evans, all made worthy by the attention she paid them. Under the intensity of her interest she harmonized everything I'd been taught to recognize as irreconcilable opposites: beauty and intelligence, nature and culture, love and benevolence, justice and goodness.

Somehow, at a moment when both my parents were shedding old friends—especially those they didn't trust enough to tell about my father's positive test and also most regretted lying to—C was let in. The summer after my first year of high school, my father drove her up to help my mother organize a concert series in Woods Hole, Massachusetts, where we'd rented a house for a few weeks. C wanted a tennis partner, and I was the only one in my family who played with any gusto. Maybe she liked that I played her to win, that I was unself-consciously showing off, unlike an older guy who would show off by trying to make her look good.

For whatever reasons, the tennis began something between us. She would bring it up with me when I failed to talk her into sleeping with me, for the first and last time, years later: "I've known you since you were fourteen, and you were the kid playing all those amazing shots at the net." It was the great taboo and the great salvation, to be held forever in that moment of a promise that I was, myself, unaware of. Back in New York, she took me to my first jazz club, invited me along to softball games with her various boyfriends, like a kind of accompanying and monitory cherub. It's easy to say now that she pitied me, or else that I was incapable of ever suspecting a genuine interest, unmixed with pity. But I felt, for the first time, a breath of openminded, hopeful concern in who I was and what I might become. I can't really explain her; she was just there.

And she was there, again, pushing back her blond hair, meeting my eyes with her flecked blue-green ones, eyes like the Afghan girl's, as we walked in a way we had of brushing arms and shoulders that was touching without touching. We went slowly down to the river, where the city vanishes; the houseboats bobbed cheerfully at anchor, gull-like, whitish gleams in the September sun, little lives that then seemed so safe and complete.

C explained that my father's threats, my mother's silent acquiescence in the use of threat, this entire mess was because they loved me and wanted me near them at the end, only they were too shy or proud to say it. I didn't need to blame myself for giving in; I'd made the right decision, without knowing it—and I shouldn't be so hard on them. What they'd done was wrong, it wasn't the best way, but behind the menace and despair there was love, which I had to see for what it was.

It would be nice to say that the sun, just then, hit the water in a particular way, a woman and her panting golden retriever jogged by, like an early messenger from a future Manhattan purged of unpleasantness; that I smiled at them, at C, at everyone; that together, not quite hand in hand, we went back to my parents' apartment, where we all forgave each other, and I helped my mother prepare dinner, set up my father's IV stand as we discussed the essays of Montaigne.

Instead, I insisted that if my father really wanted me at his side, he would have said so, not that he wanted me to study the same books he'd studied only so I could become a bitter and unfulfilled lawyer like my grandfather. In the end, however, I promised C I'd try to see my parents, to return my mother's daily phone calls. I still found it easier to think my parents meant what they said and didn't feel what they didn't say. I could not or did not want to understand that love might sometimes come dressed as aggression and fear. Better to think my parents didn't love me instead of thinking they did and were somehow bad at it . . . Better that than to think sometimes people say one thing but mean the opposite, or show their powerlessness by asserting power, that when they say, "If you don't do what I want you to do, I will cut you off," they mean, "You will never do what I want you to do, or love me as I need to be loved, and so I will take what I can get from you, even if you will hate me for it, which you do anyway."

In my anguished decision to obey what might have been my father's last wish, or rather to embrace C's interpretation of his wish, was the beginning of an acceptance of what I'd later learn to call "ordinary human misery." At the time, it was pure defeat. I'd succeeded neither in rescuing my father, nor in rebelling. I was stranded, a failure, a waste, a whistling emptiness.

For relief during those fevered days, I ran through Riverside Park, that narrow strip of meandering paths and sheltering oaks laid over the railway tunnels between the Hudson and the West Side Highway. Those paths, like so much else in Manhattan, have been so thoroughly cleaned up now that it seems scarcely believable that the Roman-style rotunda near Seventy-fourth Street, now an expensive riverfront café, once served as an unofficial homeless shelter. I jogged, or rather raced, adrenaline-filled, through the stray cats and dirty blankets hung on makeshift clotheslines, through the stink of bodies and cook fires and shopping carts piled with cans or pans, a doll, a broken chair, a guitar. The more I ran, the less I wanted to stop. I pounded on, gripped by a fear that I would eventually collapse somewhere in the labyrinth of tunnels and footpaths passing under the highway.

Worried I'd show my parents I still needed them, I made myself turn back to my narrow, long rectangle of a single room, on a floor of the Barnard campus reserved for transfer students, married Orthodox Jewish girls allowed visits from their husbands, and a group of Koreans. On weekends, they all went home noisily and happily, I thought, to parents in Brooklyn, Queens, or New Jersey. I was in the right place and not in the right place, because, although I probably should have, I did not get on the subway and go home. Instead, I put on my shorts and laced up my sneakers and went on my roundabout, pushing myself until I thought I'd fall apart. Gradually, whether because I feared or wanted the eventual injury, I stopped running altogether.

I did not want to commit suicide. Instead I felt "suicided," like a samurai who'd failed his code. But because this was America at the end of the twentieth century, no one held a sword out to me; the code itself was vague and undefined. I was not expected to do anything. And yet I sensed I was failing at that very American thing, "becoming an individual." Along with the promise of my father's money that I'd ultimately accepted, I also had to accept a reversal in what I'd once understood to be the normal order of American life. Rather than learning how to act for myself, as though I were, in every moment, colonizing a new world, I learned how to absorb, to resign, to stall. No gift is entirely free. You exchange your future for another's expectation; to take the handout is to become a part of a story that's never entirely yours, to dress yourself in the hand-me-downs of your ancestors. You take on the customs of your class, as my father had when he performed the thoroughly ritualized theater of my disinheritance, and as I would, too, someday. I also began to understand that the system or society—whatever one wants to call it—actually had a high tolerance for failure, indeed required it. A few go up, but most sink down and subside into irrelevance, stonelike or cow-like life. At every level, in neighborhoods, teams, jobs, schools and universities, there is a sorting, a sifting, or a threshing. The individual strides into his or her own over the bodies of the fallen, not even recognizing them as bodies, much as I'd plowed my way over the crisped, fallen leaves on the windy paths of Riverside Park.

I saw my parents a few times that fall, mostly at Yale–New Haven Hospital. My father was a patient there for a few days in mid-September to receive an aggressive antibiotic treatment on the cytomegalovirus that had already nearly blinded him. A series of other, smaller infections made his left eye swell shut and distorted his face. His doctors decided to insert a "shunt" above the bridge of his nose to relieve the pressure and drain the pus. He said it made him look like a rhinoceros. Another shunt had already been put into his chest so he could take the drugs without repeatedly having to pierce his skin.

It seemed they wanted to forget what had happened between us, really only a few weeks before. Nothing was mentioned about Columbia. No one apologized. Our conversation focused mainly on when my father could go home from the hospital and what might be left of him when he got there. There was still no directly life-threatening condition, no sarcoma or other cancers. But he was wasting, slowly being eaten alive after five years without a functional immune system. He was being carried off by degrees, too weak, almost, to stand, almost too weak to eat. And still he'd talk to me about the potential of the next generation of drugs in development. And then he added, "I won't make it that long," and, "Don't worry, I won't become a vegetable either."

Shortly after Thanksgiving, he felt pain of uncertain origin. The only thing that could stop it, for a time, was Demerol, which my father recognized as the beginning of a cascade toward semi-consciousness. After Demerol would come morphine, and, after morphine, either prolonged coma or death. He wasn't about to find out which. The pain lessened for a day, two days, and then returned. At night, he began to take the morphine.

The following Friday morning, the phone rang in my room. I was hoping it was the girl from the summer, whom I'd been struggling not to call. She'd broken up with her boyfriend, or else he with her. The story wasn't clear. I'd begun walking her home from the library after my job at the bookstore, where I'd kept working in case my father decided to go ahead and disinherit me anyway. One night, in an unusual reversal, she'd come to meet me at the store and walked me back to my room, where we talked and smoked awkwardly out the window, gradually falling silent before she abruptly said she had to go finish an assignment. She left her pack of cigarettes, which I immediately set out to return, either afraid I'd smoke them all at once or because I'd sensed a pretext. She'd sent me home at sunrise, before her suitemates could wake and notice the stranger emerging from their common bathroom. We'd been seeing each other almost every night since, sometimes reading together until we fell asleep, but had agreed to take a week off because exams were coming up and papers were due. Hoping that she'd given in and called me first, I could not, at first, recognize my mother's voice on the line. "I think this is it," she said. "You'd better come."

My father greeted me from the white couch, a swirling silk paisley dressing gown in reds and golds worn over his powder-blue boxers and white T-shirt. That day's *Times* was on the glass coffee table, face up, unopened. "You're sure?" I asked him, which was what he asked me before I resigned a chess game. I couldn't think of what else to say. He was sure, he said. "Sodium cyanide," he explained, "can take you one of two ways. When it enters the heart it causes almost immediate cardiac arrest, a heart attack. Everything stops. If your heart muscle is relaxed, then it's a very peaceful death; they say painless. If your heart is pumping blood out and contracted, then the body goes into a seizure. It's a fifty-fifty chance."

"Do you want me to stay?" I asked.

"No, no, don't stay. They might arrest you."

"For what?"

"You can't kill yourself in this country. It's illegal."

I hugged him, which it seemed I hadn't done for years. One of my arms could now reach almost entirely around his torso. I feared breaking something. Someone was trembling. I couldn't think of anything to say. Nothing was said. "I'll miss you," I came out with, finally, which was again a borrowed line; it was what my girlfriend had started saying to me instead of "I love you," which neither of us could yet tell the other, or maybe "I miss you" was closer to the truth.

"I miss my mother every day," my father said. His last words to me.

I went out and waited on the black sofa in the music room. Motionless, I looked out the windows as I'd done so often, staring at the skeletal branches still hung with tattered leaves and a stray wind-whipped plastic bag. A small eternity passed, and my mother called out to me. "Don't go in," she said. I went in. Smell of shit. Mouth fixed open in a grimace of pain. Legs curled fetally. One hand outstretched, another in a fist. A seizure. I went out. Later, my father's remaining friend and colleague from the hematology department came to say goodbye before the ambulance men arrived from the funeral home. I was surprised ambulances were still required for dead people. The paramedics, or whatever they were called, handed me my father's glasses as they bundled him onto the stretcher and out the door. I went back into the room. The dressing gown had been folded carefully and placed on a chair. On the table, a glass of water, the newspaper. I went out. I went in. I sat on the couch. I sipped from the glass of water. I put it back.

Without really thinking about it, I began to read the *Times*: The head of the Medellín cocaine cartel had been killed in Colombia, former Soviet munitions workers faced poverty as their plants closed down, President Bill Clinton had convened a special panel to examine existing welfare laws, Mayor-elect Rudy Giuliani had appointed William Bratton as police commissioner, the weather for the next day would be cloudy, with highs in the 50s, rain, heavy at times, tapering off toward nightfall.

The words flooded over me in a black-and-white hum. When I put down the paper, my sweating hands and palms were grimed with print. There would be another edition and another, day after day, world without end, in which, every day, smaller worlds were extinguished, never to appear again. I had pictured this moment of his death so many times that when it actually came it felt dreamlike, something I'd remembered before it actually happened, a photograph that had leaped from a page of those once-forbidden German volumes. I stayed there, a thinking stone, until it was time to go to the funeral home.

The next morning, my mother and I, along with my father's sister and her husband, followed a hearse out of Riverside Memorial Chapel, up the Henry Hudson Parkway to the cemetery— Westchester Hills, they called it, although it was closer to traditionally working-class Yonkers, not "middle-class" Westchester. We stood silently in the early winter rain, watching as the coffin was winched down into a neat rectangular gash in the steep hillside overlooking the Hudson. It was a plain coffin my mother and I had picked out the day before, in Riverside Memorial's basement showroom, to the obvious disappointment of the salesman. The dirt resounded dully against the pine as each of us poured a shovelful of clotted and stony earth onto the lid. That was it: almost exactly as my father wanted. My mother carried out his instructions practically to the letter—no service, no prayer for the dead, no eulogies, no guests. My aunt's husband was allowed to attend only after a brief argument my mother lacked the energy to maintain: no friends, no extended family, not even my cousins, the perfect girls my father had so much admired.

After a few minutes of standing around, the other three returned to the warmth of the hired car. I continued to shovel from the prepared pile as the official grave-diggers looked on. I would have done it all day, to the end, unused even as I was to this kind of work. My palms split open after about two minutes. The rain and cold had hardened the soil into great, rocky clumps. It felt more like carving than digging. But what did I know? Did I think it would be like filling in a sand pit on a beach? I sensed the cemetery men cocking eyebrows at each other as I struggled for traction on the slope. I wondered if they'd seen this sort of thing before. The families who could afford Westchester Hills were not likely to have spent much time among shovels. I jabbed into the pile; one black wingtip pushing down on the top of the shovel blade, the way I must have seen it done in movies, and I came up with more than I could lift, broke the slabs into manageable pieces, stopped, removed my coat and jacket, and stood in a dress shirt I probably had to throw away, shoveling, spattering mud onto my black jeans until my mother came out of the car to tell me that the grave-diggers' union required them to fill in most of the grave. It could have been a lie, but I accepted it dumbly. A higher power, of a sort, had at last intervened. Who was I to protest against the organization of death workers? I retreated to the limousine, bleeding hands in my pockets, where we watched one of them plow a small bulldozer into the mound, finishing in a few mechanical minutes what would have taken me an eternity. Then, to my humiliation, the men smoothed the surface and we drove off.

Our family lawyer, a former colleague of my grandfather, read out the will in our living room, a week later. I received about $600,000 in various stocks and treasuries. My mother received an equal amount, plus whatever she could get from the sale of our Central Park West duplex apartment. A hospital for torture victims in Denmark was the other beneficiary.

If some friend, or even my mother, had asked me then what I felt about all this, I wouldn't have known what to say. I was deeply delighted, in an old, eighteenth-century sense of that word, when it used to describe the feeling of a great weight removed. For the previous five years, my father had been sick and dying, without hope of recovery. For most of my childhood, before that, beginning when I was about six, he'd been subject to accidents and multiple ailments: two dislocated shoulders from falling in the street, a chronically bad back, a serious bout of hepatitis B he'd caught at the same time he'd become infected with HIV. The afternoon of his death, I remembered the last line of Kafka's *Metamorphosis*, after Gregor Samsa has been swept out with the garbage and the family goes for a walk in Prague's open air. For the first time, the story leaves the confines of the Samsa apartment. Magically, it is springtime. Gregor's sister, so long in the shadows, "sprang to her feet first and stretched her young body."

That stretching brings with it a great feeling of justice, for Gregor's sister had been the only one who really cared for him after his transformation and brief life as an insect. But that emotion had no place, and could not take place for me. There was nothing I could say I'd done for my father. I'd ruined his last months with all the stupidity about college. I was glad not to be disinherited but I intended to give all the money away immediately.

I went up the stairs and into my old room, almost untouched since I'd last slept there. I sat at my old desk in front of an Apple II computer nobody had thrown away, hands poised over the control, apple, and reset keys. Books from the summer, still un-packed, were laid out on the bed, waiting for my emancipation. I smoked out the window, looking down Sixty-ninth Street, won-dering what my father would want me to do. The answer was that I must do what I always had done, which was carry on as though nothing had happened.

I wandered off down the hall into my parents' bedroom, as I'd walked down the hall as a child, awakened by nightmares. Sometimes, noticing a light through the transom and thinking it was morning, I would set off to wake my parents, only to find my father was in bed, reading or listening to music, and I had scarcely slept at all. I forget how young I was when I first learned always to knock, or how I learned that lesson. I walked in bewildered, checking to see if he was there, checking to see if he was still not there.

I searched his dressing table, not sure what I'd find, not sure even what I was looking for. The morphine tablets were right next to the pillow, but I didn't really want them for myself. I wanted something tangible and permanent. I searched the drawers, perhaps hoping he'd left me a secret letter, his real will. I moved on to the clothes closet. His ties still trailed off the in-side doorknob, as if waiting to be worn to work. They must have been like that for months. I looked through them, finding noth-ing that pleased me in the broad 1970s stripes. My father had terrible taste in ties, almost deliberately bad. He hated them, he said to me once, but he'd worn them to school every day since he'd been in first grade and he felt undressed without them. A few weeks later, my mother and I were going through the closet together and found a few shirts neither of us had seen him wear, two lumberjack plaids, but of a fine cotton, a burgundy Pierre Cardin linen shirt, a finely woven Perry Ellis rainbow-striped oxford. These I started wearing around.

One thing I did take with me from my search: a cassette recording of Henry Purcell's seventeenth-century proto-opera, *Dido and Aeneas*. The tape was lying amid a stack of others on the bedside table. There were, in fact, stacks and heaps everywhere, of old journals and magazines on the broad, benchlike radiator cover, clothes on a rocking chair. It was like an obvious visual pun: "Things had indeed been piling up for the Roth family, lately." I pocketed the tape, then, without really knowing why, although I knew that *Dido and Aeneas* was the occasion of one of the only times my father showed any emotion to me at all.

I'd walked in on him, without knocking, one night, around the end of my last year of high school. I don't know when or for what. I probably wanted something that must have seemed immensely important. I wasn't exactly terrified of approaching him, but I was wary of asking for anything, like whether he would come to see me in our school's production of *Macbeth*, or listen to my orchestra concert. He'd already begun removing himself from my life, perhaps out of courtesy or delicacy of feeling— would I really want to have to introduce this gaunt, shuffling man as my father to my cruel classmates?—or maybe he was training me for his too-soon total disappearance. Yet I took it as rejection. The pain on his face when I brought these things up was the pain that flickered when he heard a false note or someone coughed too loudly at a concert or I slammed a door in the apartment. The orchestra might play out of tune or out of tempo; as for *Macbeth*, as much as I insisted it was still fucking Shakespeare and the production really excellent, I had only a series of minor roles, barely speaking parts. The director had made us stop shaving and grow out our hair. In a cast photograph, I look like a character from some Russian novel, muttonchop sideburns, an old country peasant.

There was music coming from a boombox. Over a restrained dirge from the strings, a woman singing in minor key, her voice rising and falling in waves meant to imitate the breath of the dying:

When I am laid, am laid in earth
May my wrongs create no trouble, no trouble in thy breast.
Remember me, remember me, but forget my fate.

I listened in the doorway, unnoticed. My father was crying. He sensed me and called out, "Turn it off. I can't bear it." I walked in and pressed STOP. My father blew his nose and, to gather himself, asked if I knew the story from the *Aeneid*.

I couldn't think what led my father to identify himself with the mythical queen of Carthage who'd killed herself when abandoned by her beloved Aeneas, as he sailed off to found Rome. I did not question it at all. It seemed perfectly natural to me that music or literature was a kind of mirror of the self. One could be Dido dying, or Kafka's sister, or even murderous Macbeth. They fitted themselves to you or you to them. I didn't think it grandiose, or even perverse, that my father, whose life had been absurdly altered by a too-casual slip of a needle, could think of himself as a figure of high tragedy. "Remember me, but forget my fate." That was the command I, too, would obey. Our tiny Carthage would go on.

5

My mother said she had no use for me around the apartment. She wouldn't sell it for months. There was nothing to be done, no visits to expect. Happy to be spared what seemed like idle and empty waiting, I ducked back into the subway and roared uptown to the neoclassical façades and chattering students of Columbia. I began writing my paper on the late-nineteenth-century French poet Stéphane Mallarmé. Going on meant I had to finish my work for the semester. It was what had always been expected of me.

Mallarmé's collected poems begin like this: "Nothing, this residue, virgin verse." In my single dorm room, I delved into this icy, mysterious poetry, full of tricky grammatical inversions and overturned clichés. Mallarmé set me adrift on the ocean of language, as he does all his readers. We are a vessel shipwrecked, without masts to give purposeful motion, yet somehow it's the sailors who sing and the sirens who drown.

A poetry of poetry, much of the time the verses verged on nonsense or music. Rich with noises I could barely understand, like *"Aboli bibelot d'inanité sonore,"* it was also full of abolitions, nothings, haunted by its own will to nothingness. "A toss of the dice will never abolish chance," goes the tonic chord of his most famous work, a work written like a musical score, with overlapping lines in different typefaces, able to be read all at once or sideways, up and down as well as left to right. That poem ends with a sentence in a dwindling, diminuendo typeface proclaiming that "nothing will take place but the place, except perhaps a constellation."

Fixing on such an abstract distraction with the earth still brown and raw on my father's grave was surprisingly easy. Mallarmé's music, nonsense, silence, and coldness all felt impersonally personal. Before the glowing azure blank of my computer screen, I struggled with this new idea that art could be quite useless or meaningless, that language would do its own thing, if left to its own devices, that the poet and the reader must learn to get their consciousness, their shaping power, out of the way, to let writing run its course, just as, say, the processes of protein synthesis ran their course in varying patterns, broken off and copied from the master text.

That winter's first snowfall silted down as words filled the screen. After the snow, it rained hard for a day. Overnight the temperature suddenly dropped well below freezing. The sidewalks were coated in ice; a hard crust formed over the park paths. Without footholds, we skated down the streets in even the hardiest boots, whipped along by the wind.

I ran into a classmate from our French poetry class coming out of Butler Library. D was bone thin, muffled in layers of sweaters against the cold. I'd always liked what he said in class, liked the way I never seemed to see him speaking to anyone else, much as I barely spoke to anyone. We nodded to each other. "It snows in the city as it snows in our hearts," I said to him. He smiled, and reminded me that it was only an accident of nature; we mustn't indulge the pathetic fallacy, he said. Nature did not exist to reflect our moods, it mocked us with meaning. The actual numbness we felt had nothing to do with the fact that D knew himself to be frozen in the body of a thirteen-year-old, after an adolescent thyroid tumor had wrecked his hormones, or that I was, once again, a glacial waste, even more so since my girlfriend had dumped me two weeks after my father's death and started hanging out with a sports editor from the college newspaper. I ought not to have blamed her. I was no fun at all, and her college program did not include taking care of the grieving. I probably frightened her out of her wits; too much, too soon. The gaping grave was inside me, too.

"We must remember," D said consolingly, as we skated into a Chinese restaurant, "that we are pure critical intelligence."

I was about to fall or had already fallen under the spell of what the academic shorthand of the time called Theory. No particular professor or class led me to it so much as Theory wrapped me in an entire climate of description. I'm sure my old shrink would have pointed out that I'd found one area of knowledge my father seemed to have missed entirely. Then, I knew only that Theory was simply, shoulder-shruggingly, the only thing that helped me to see what I was and where.

The word *theory* meant a lot of different things to a lot of different people. Both its opponents and apostles appeared to agree that it was, according to one pro-theory professor, "the post-Enlightenment critique of humanism and the Enlightenment." In the words of another, it was "the persistent critique of what we cannot not inhabit." This last definition made instant sense to me, despite the typically baroque language Theory's advocates were always attacked for using. It was like going to Columbia University without really wanting to be there and without a better alternative, because no matter which way you turned, someone was harmed. There was no opting out.

Critics made a lot out of how incomprehensible Theory was, how it masked its writers' confusions by trying to make the reader run through a labyrinth of proper names—Hegel, Marx, Kierkegaard, Benjamin, Foucault, Bataille, Adorno, de Man, and technical concepts such as sublation, species being, the aesthetic, the mass, the aura, the local focus of power, *différance*, metalepsis, anamorphosis, catechresis. Through it all, however, I began to notice a clear tendency: "Man" as the measure of all things, "the human form divine," the reasoner, the maker of meanings, was not really so centrally important after all. We were all governed by deep forces, large and small, all beyond our control, forces such as language, desire, economics, evolution. "Man" or "human being" was just a name for the weak vessel that bore us ceaselessly into the future, and that name, too, was about to be discarded. According to the essays D and I inhaled bit by bit, night after night, the very idea that there was such a thing as "man" was rapidly being liquidated, or had already been liquidated. " 'Man' is but a figure in the sand, washed away by the incoming tides": thus spake Michel Foucault in 1967.

To me, these words felt like accurate descriptions of the world I was already living in and had no choice but to go on through. It seemed tragic, to live through this disappearance of an earlier ideal of the self, as one might sit at the bedside of a dying family member. A true theorist might say that I was merely learning to let go of myself as an active first person, an effective "I," and that I, or whatever took the place of that I, might be better off for accepting the loss.

Theory also seemed to suggest that in the constant struggle to better oneself or others, we were as likely to make things worse. For every recent improvement in the human condition there was a corresponding horror, invisible furies rising up to punish us for our pride. Dignified man had invented the atomic bomb, killed millions in wars and planned purges, enslaved millions more. For every amelioration there was a corresponding pollution, a pollution often greater than the improvement. "The fully enlightened earth radiates disaster triumphant." This was a slogan and a sentiment I could get behind. After all, my fully enlightened family had been nothing but a disaster.

Time passed to this drumbeat of doom in the back of my consciousness. A spring thaw came, the students spilled out of their dorms into the sun. Dressed up or stripped down, they co-agulated into a mass of naked arms and legs, a Frisbee flashed through the air, music played, and the sky shimmered with little waves of giddiness. This was the real contemporary civilization, more than the required core courses all Columbia students had to take, but I could not stretch myself to meet it. Fun was other people.

Neither could I find myself among the groups who pitched their tents along the college walk connecting the Broadway and Amsterdam gates: the young Republicans, the Asian Students Association, the Students of Color Association, the student government, the Campus Crusade for Christ, the Sparticist League, Students for Israel, Students for Palestine, the premed study-break tent, some team or other racing past in their bright baby-blue jackets. I couldn't understand everyone's eagerness to participate in something, to yoke themselves to the same traditions and pastimes that could only lead to repeating the same unhappiness later on. If that was supposed to be life, I was against it. Yet how could anyone be against life? Wasn't I just against lives that seemed so self-assured, so perfectly and pragmatically planned?

Part of what Theory promised, beyond the suspicious questioning of human agency and motive, was an idea that another world was still possible, not in some mythical afterlife, but on this earth, now, that the life around me did not have to be the only one. There was no fixed human nature except to take in and shape what was around us. And almost everything around us was now the result of some kind of human endeavor, like the soy formula I'd been nursed on. We were culture and artificiality and engineering all the way down. What was made could thus be remade.

Theory's other saving power was that it required a lot of close and busy work. D and I would meet in the library or in the off-campus apartment he shared with his sister, a law student, on 113th Street, and go over our notes. We quizzed each other: What is a sign and what is a referent? Where is the ambiguity in sonnet 116? We'd eat Korean food and report on our reading. D would pull out a book with a glossy, nearly neon-green cover from his

satchel, and, letting his hands glide along the spine in a way that
mingled salaciousness and pedantry, open it to the first essay,
"The Resistance to Theory," by Paul de Man. Then he'd pass it
to me, pointing to an underlined passage. I read aloud, "The resistance to theory is the resistance to reading . . ."

D took this in between slurps of his fish-head hot pot. He
always was eager to try things on the menu that would lead the
waiter to explain, without actually saying the words, that they
were not meant for "white people." "The encounter with the other
must be absolute," D pronounced when the dish arrived. Then,
in his hometown Memphis accent, no less faked for being his native city's, "but it kind of does smell like ass."

And, later, when we asked ourselves why we were studying
all of this when we could have been premed, or preparing for law
school, careers in politics or finance, we stumbled onto this one,
"Literature as well as criticism . . . is condemned (or privileged)
to be forever the most rigorous and, consequently, the most unreliable language in terms of which man names and transforms
himself." D and I delighted in these paradoxes: the most rigorous and therefore the most unreliable, names and, by naming,
transforms. The deeper we went, the less certain we were. Our
confusion was like a sign of progress. Aiming for the essence of
literature or of the human, our work just exposed what we lacked,
a lack that could never be filled, was not supposed to be filled
but, rather, in a perverse way, "enjoyed."

We were very good at this kind of enjoyment. One book led
to another, one critic to another critic of that critic. The game
kept us alive and made it easy for us not to think about those
other absences in our own lives: my father, D's thyroid.

We agreed with the French philosopher-psychoanalyst team
Gilles Deleuze and Félix Guattari that the importance of families was overstated. Our causes and conditions lay outside them.
So, too, our desires, which floated fractal-like, barely coherent:
the small, shell-like ear of that girl from the French department,

lobe lit by the winter sunset through the western window of the seminar room, the honeyed smile of the Ethiopian coffee-shop waitress and the way she had of saying your name when she brought you your order, the Indian premed in a faux leopardskin coat who always left some iced drink behind her when she got up from lecture, a perfect imprint of lipstick on the straw.

Framed in the window of that Broadway Korean joint, D, his face gaunt, both too old and too young for a twenty-year-old, topped with round tortoiseshell glasses, his parted hair and stiffly collared shirts looking like he'd stepped from a photograph album of turn-of-the-century Irish intellectuals, me trying to sketch one of Deleuze's "schizo-diagrams" in the air with a pair of chopsticks, we probably appeared to be political activists of some outmoded Marxist sect, or lovers. I actually wore a beret; I'd found it at the flea market on Seventy-sixth Street and Columbus Avenue. It was the only kind of hat that I could pack my curly hair into, or so I told myself and anyone who asked. I referred to it as my hairnet, and sometimes even wore it in class.

At least one person thought the beret was a quiet way of announcing I was sexually confused. But he thought everyone who wasn't already gay was sexually confused. He was an activist in the campus's Lesbian, Gay, Bisexual, Transgender organization, and lived down the hall from me in a shared suite—I'd finally moved to a small room in a dorm meant for the "artsy types." He'd even dyed his hair pink. His camped-up, queeny voice broadcast down the corridor unceasingly; he was usually on the phone arguing, and his arguments were spectacular performances, always quivering on the edge of outrage and offense, even when planning an action, gossiping, or holding court in his room to an apparently constant stream of guests. "*I* have to keep an open-door policy," he said one night, after he came into my room and surprisingly slammed the door behind him. "You're not my type," he told me, "but we'll find you a nice boy. If you like nice boys." I suppose I might even have played along a bit. I signed the

petitions he dropped off under my door, and, once, on my way
back from the shower, in my bathrobe, went into his room. He
had to show me something, he said, but I could have easily told
him I'd get dressed first. I was being provocatively indifferent, or
perhaps curious to see what he'd do. I went to the LGBT rave,
where he pressed two tabs of what turned out to be acid into my
hand.

I took one and gave the other to the girl who'd once wanted
to see me again in the fall of what seemed another life. We were
back together, and still missing each other. We looked at the lights
on the Harlem side of Morningside Park. They grew brighter,
shinier, pulsated like stars, and then they began to go out. We
walked back to her room, the way we used to. We would miss each
other forever. She began to cry, and I found myself comforting her
until it seemed suddenly that the effort of holding her was too
much. "I just don't have a body anymore. I miss my body," I said.
She missed her body, too. We wept for our missing bodies. "Do
you think this is what it's like to be dead?" we asked each other.
We thought it probably was as close as we'd come to knowing.
Toward morning, we fell asleep, encircled in our puppet arms. We
awoke in the afternoon, slowly ourselves; a pain in the base
of our spines from the strychnine-laced acid welcomed us back
to life. I'd failed to become "pure critical intelligence," at least
that way.

As the end of college neared, I decided it would be unethical
to apply for any of the university fellowships, not that I thought
I stood much chance of them. I reasoned they were intended for
people who needed the money. I no longer needed the money.
Other classmates who also needed money or wanted money were
going to law school, or joining investment banks, or heading off
to Silicon Valley to invent cyborgs. My girlfriend had already
graduated and had gone off on a research fellowship. They had
got what they came to college for, the degree, the passport to success. But what had I gone to college for? I couldn't really say, un-

less it was to master "the persistent critique of what I cannot not inhabit."

I awarded myself a grant from what I privately dubbed the Eugene Roth, Jr., Memorial Scholarship Fund: $60,000 to go to Paris and continue my studies with Jacques Derrida, one of the grand masters of a theory of language and personality that grew out of Mallarmé's ideas about poetry. Derrida's work emphasized the accidental, the exceptional, the perverse. It, too, was haunted by a sense of absence, of life lived in the perpetual presence of death, of death as the foundation of philosophy. In the best So-cratic tradition, Derrida seemed to be saying—and I could never be quite sure in fact what he was saying—that philosophy was about "learning how to die."

My decision even seemed like something my father would have approved of, or at least been incapable of disapproving. I'd gone all the way on to the end, though I did miss the actual grad-uation ceremony, my cornea having somehow gotten scratched the night before. D and I had gone out and toasted our futures a few too many times at the Night Café. My eyes, the doctor ex-plained, were all dried out.

This last lapse, too, it seemed my father would not have minded, since he always said he hated "Pomp and Circumstance," both the march and the things themselves. Better "Remember me, but forget my fate." Not much difference in his mind between a graduation and a funeral; not much difference in my own mind either. I lay in my old four-poster bed, which had been my mother's, in her new, smaller apartment on West End Avenue and 104th Street, my left eye, the better of my two nearsighted ones, watering uncontrollably. The spring sun glinted off the windows of the nearby buildings and threw strange, looming shadows on the apartment's still bare white walls. For a moment, I worried that these blotches were now a permanent part of my vision, that I'd have to get used to looking at the world through them, like a poorly adjusted microscope. I thought I could hear my father's voice: "When you look into the microscope, you will see the outline of a red cell, and, in the center, the blue twists, those are the malaria parasites. If you move the slide around, as I showed you, you'll see some of the cells are almost bursting with blue. Those parasites will burst out of the cell and move on."

I believed I was also ready to move on. My mother made no objections to my Paris project: she was already talking about coming to visit, once I'd got installed, and how I should be sure to call my father's friends there and see if they could find me an apartment. I told her I'd send her a postcard with my new address, once I had one, and I had no intention of calling the family friends. My father's death hadn't turned us into a tightly knit family of two. While I'd been uptown in college, she'd been driving the New Jersey Turnpike to help take care of her stroke-ridden father in suburban Philadelphia. She did this while establishing a career of her own, providing young musicians with the opportunities and support she'd never had or failed to take when presented.

She liked to say she was a "good carer," but, to my annoyance, it seemed she was most comfortable where such practiced caring took place at either the most basic level of human survival or in helping the already confident advance their careers. I had no doubt that were I to collapse suddenly, to find myself crippled or overdosed, my mother would run to me as though I were still the five-year-old who'd skinned his knee, just as she would have been proud of me if I'd done anything she could have been proud of. But the greater part of life between suffering and success seemed to elude her, at least when it came to me. There had been much of everyday family life my mother and I had seemed to miss. I'd grown up without her, even though she'd been there most of the time while I was growing up.

It also seemed that she wanted something from me that was as total and absolute as what she gave to others. I wasn't sure what that was, exactly, but it made me want to run away. Mostly, she wanted me to accept her frequent offers to accompany her to concerts and movies, her invitations to tête-à-tête dinners on Jewish holidays that she didn't otherwise observe, her phone calls in which she talked about my grandparents' increasingly doomed health with the kind of dry, medical precision she'd learned by listening to my father talk about the progress of his disease. Sometimes she'd call me up to tell me about the success of her latest musician protégées—they were always women—the state of the Clinton administration, her latest coincidental run-in with a former classmate's parent, or a family friend I hadn't seen since I was four.

These relentlessly one-way conversations, seeming to hint at some common life she thought we'd shared, reduced me to a seething silence I knew how to break only by some terrific act of rage, as though every one of our conversations brought me back to the dish cupboard, the neatly stacked plates that had appeared to insult me with their innocent orderliness. My mother seemed to be performing an elaborate evasion under cover of reaching out to me, but I couldn't say what she was evading. I was unable to forgive her for not taking my side when my father was threatening to disinherit me, but I also felt rottenly juvenile for remaining hurt. My mother seemed to have buried the incident with my father and never mentioned it.

Before I left for Paris, later that August, I copied into my notebook a line attributed to Kierkegaard that I'd found in Harold Bloom's *The Anxiety of Influence*, "The one who works will give birth to his own father." At the time, I took it to mean that fatherless as I now was, I must forget the father I'd had in order to find, within myself, the one who would actually let me go without cutting me off first. Where to start that work, I had no idea. And before starting, I thought, I would have to learn how to live, which was why people like me went to Paris in the first place: to live.

6

In Paris, I died young and died often. In the local open-air market, jostled from behind by one of the basket-wielding old women eager for Friday fish, I was thrust onto a marlin's spike and disemboweled; I slipped on one of the ubiquitous dog turds and bashed my temple on the curb, or on one of the city's irregular cobblestones: coma, curtains; I fell out the window of my apartment while craning for a view of the Pantheon at sunset; stealing a look up the billowing skirt of a sexy bicyclist, I was run over by a bus, or the *belle cycliste* coming at me—more and more naked inner thigh shown with each pedal push, until she appeared gloriously, revolutionarily *sans culottes*, or *déculottée*—she knocked me into the path of an oncoming car; my irritable water heater exploded, mid-shower, scalding me to death; the apartment's old electric radiator short-circuited, scattering sparks on the pea-green shag carpet, which burned like an oil slick; I choked on a stale baguette. I noted these all down on a postcard to D, on a fellowship at Cambridge. "The book of ignominious deaths," I called it, while I imagined how, on my way to the mail, I'd trip on the spiral stairs, in the dark, reaching for the light's timer.

These various fantasies of my early and absurd demise were stirrings, probably not the first, of a private theology of accident that came to govern my time in Paris—as if the only way to give any meaning to the meaninglessness I felt was to find new ways to affirm that random, unanticipated events made up life's only valid kind of meaning. I was ready to believe that any rational structure I tried to give myself, my disciplined reading of French novels in the public libraries, for instance, would be undermined by a much deeper structure, a law of chaos, that would always interrupt me at the moment I felt most in control of my fate. At any moment, I thought, my life could be changed forever, in ways I couldn't possibly prepare for. Alongside the quotation from Bloom's book about work and giving birth to one's own father, I'd also copied out another one: "It was a great marvel that they were in the father without knowing him." I put the two opposed quotations side by side, as if they might magically react with each other and reveal something, the way that photography had been discovered by leaving a piece of silver-nitrate-coated paper out in the sun, and then forgot about them.

I was waiting for Derrida, but his seminar was not supposed to begin until October. I'd arrived in August, the vacation month, when the city empties out and only tourist spots remain open. The few remaining Parisians seemed to keep to themselves, floating along the boulevards on bicycles or clacking quickly along narrow streets before vanishing behind thick wooden doors and into hidden courtyards. Or perhaps they, too, like me, longed to escape. I'd arrived in a city of fantasists who dreamed of starting their lives again elsewhere, as I'd dreamed of starting mine over in their city. Even in Paris, there was always another Paris to escape to.

I fell in with a Lebanese kid, Saamer Saad, I'd crossed paths with a few times at Columbia. We ran into each other, or rather he picked me up, one day when I'd taken my notebook and a copy of Baudelaire's prose poems to one of the anonymous chain cafés behind the Place du Panthéon, a small oval I usually avoided because it was heavily trafficked by foreign students, like me, tourists, Aussie backpackers, Americans in college sweatshirts. I'd been there a while, unable to concentrate, listening to the babble of languages, the defeated diphthongs of atrocious French, "Shah view-dray unh Coca light," when Saamer swung suddenly into a wicker chair, grabbed the Baudelaire off the table, and began to page through it.

That grab was typical. He later boasted of how he had no fear of making a bad impression, even courted it. He told me how, at Columbia, he'd picked out girls from families that still held to traditional ideas of marriage and virginity—Indians, Chinese, Midwestern Christians, never other Arabs, he said—who wanted sex terribly but forced him to play seducer. He had to satisfy their desire to be victims of someone else's desire. And yet he'd grown bored of that game, he said. He'd come to Paris without any specific plan except to not be in medical school, where his father, a former general in the Lebanese army, wanted him. Short and taut, with brown eyes shining with near-yellow light, he blended in my mind with an image I had of Julien Sorel, the anti-hero of Stendhal's novel *The Red and the Black*, a would-be Napoléon who comes of age only after Napoléon's fall, trapped in a reactionary moment of conformity and boring careerism. This sense of resemblance increased when he told me how, as he was crossing the old wooden-planked pedestrian bridge that linked the Louvre to the old Mint, he felt what he described as an obligation to jump onto one of the tourist boats passing underneath. He'd made it, but had nearly been arrested by the police and declared a terrorist, before convincing them he was just a drunk tourist. This kind of willed recklessness linked to his stories of forced seduction and reminded me of a scene in the novel when Julien decides he must try to hold hands with his employer's wife at a dinner party, not because he knows he's in love with her, but because his idea of life seems to require him to seduce her.

After our first meeting, Saamer began to come around to my apartment. He'd lock himself out of his own repeatedly, as though he had an allergy to keys, or perhaps to memory. He'd turn up at late hours wanting to borrow my camera, or money, since his parents had cut him off until he agreed to go become a doctor.

At first, I gave in willingly to his requests. His case seemed a less complicated echo of my own, and I was curious to see whether he'd make a more successful bid for his freedom than I'd done. Also, I was glad for his interruptions, which made up my only human contact apart from the characters in the French novels I read through with a half-distracted diligence, dictionary at my elbow, a notebook at hand, a pencil in my mouth as much as it was in my hand, aware sometimes that I was merely letting time pass, turning pages, lost in the *inanité sonore*.

He asked me once if I ever wrote anything or just read. I laughed uneasily. Secretly, I often wrote, but had nothing really to show for it. It felt shameful and clichéd. I'd been drafting a scene, a parable about a boy who, walking down a medieval street in an old European city, leans against a wall. The wall, under the pressure of the boy's hand, begins to dissolve to reveal the history of its construction, the serfs who worked on it, the lives of the prostitutes who solicited in its shadow, the plague victims who died at its feet, the family of Jews who lived on its other side. I was trying to come to terms with Paris as a city that had so far repeatedly repulsed my advances to know it, even as I could pretend to know what was going on, like the dream apartment I'd visited as a child.

Under different circumstances, my friendship with Saamer might have been short-lived. I felt he used up all the air in the room, like a raging fire. I felt caught, too, in this tandem he'd created, in which I was meant to be the responsible, grown-up one. It felt familiarly oppressive to me, but I couldn't say why. As if sensing my impatience and unease, although his real reason soon became apparent, he stayed away for a few weeks before he called to say he wanted to introduce me to a friend.

The woman I came to think of as "Helen of Troy" was the daughter of a Lebanese poet, an art school friend of Saamer's roommate. My father might have seen her as the particularly bountiful outcome of Levantine genetic mixing: Greeks from the

time of Alexander the Great, Arabs, Crusaders, Ottomans—
themselves a mix of Macedonian Greeks, Turks from the steppes,
and original Trojans. DNA recognized only the recombination of
patterns, differences in generational repetitions, but I imagined
the woman who'd walked in an hour late to our rendezvous was
what that ancient prince, the one who gave his name to the city
where we met, must have seen when, arriving at last in mythic
Sparta, he claimed the reward for having chosen love over wisdom
and power.

Around her hung a scent of hidden loss as narcotically at-
tractive to me as her waves of black hair, her green-flecked brown
eyes in a face that seemed sculpted by someone who still believed
in the old Greek gods. We were hanging out one night in her
apartment in the ultramodern suburb of La Défense—Saamer,
Helen, and I—a little after they'd fallen in love. They'd just
adopted a kitten. The kitten was testing its claws, its bite, on
Saamer's bare arm. I was looking out the window onto the extremely un-Parisian view of blinking red lights, poised atop slum-
bering office towers, great black shapes against the darkness lit
only by airplanes making their approach overhead. Helen joined
me at the window.

"I remember when I was about three years old," she said, "in
Beirut. We lived in a tall, modern apartment building. When the
war started, at night, you could see the tracer shells, the mortars
in the sky. I adored watching them. They were beautiful to me,
then. My sister always had to come and take me away from the
windows, down to the shelter. But I always adored them. I could
not be frightened. I think, perhaps, this is my problem."

"Fucking monster," Saamer said, laughing, as he stood up,
raised his arm in the air, bright lines of blood appearing where
the kitten, still holding tight, was pulling itself up onto him with
its baby claws.

For a while, we went almost everywhere together, in a trio:
movies, restaurants, clubs. "She likes it," Saamer said, when I

thought I might be annoying them, "it keeps us from fighting." But I didn't really keep them from fighting. I was more like a witness than a referee. They had tremendous shouting matches in Arabic, then made up on the spot, wrestling, giggling, biting, while I slipped away, promising myself to go back to my books, to the unfinished parable about the wall, and my research. We were together without rivalry, loneliness, restlessness, or fear.

Derrida's seminar "On Hospitality" began, at last, in November. This was the moment I'd been waiting for. I was determined to meet the man, to shake the hand of this shadow of some unseen power of intellectual greatness. Someone said he rarely showed up for his office hours at the free university where he gave his public classes, but I tracked him down, and was there on the right day, outside a small orange-carpeted office, an hour early and third in line.

At college we used to say he looked like God, but when I got through, at last, I thought he looked like a long-lost North African cousin of my grandfather, or even, with his great white mane and jutting chin, a bit like my father's sister. He wore clumsy tortoiseshell reading glasses and moved nervously, playing with a pipe on his desk. The office was bare, standard office-supply desk and chairs, his coat and leather briefcase. He seemed uncomfortable in it. I felt at home: that is, I felt terrified in an utterly familiar way, as though my father were about to ask me whether I'd asked a good question in school. I had written "Marco Roth, étudiant américain de Columbia University" on the secretary's sheet and he was holding it when I came in. He asked me about Columbia, about the professor there he'd known, about my plans in Paris with perfunctory disinterest and in a way that made it seem I'd showed up at his door by chance, or on a whim, just like that. It was impossible for me to admit that he was pretty much my entire plan in Paris.

The seminar really turned out to be a lecture. The room was an amphitheater and usually not more than half filled. We met every two or three weeks (depending on the master's frequent travel schedule) for three or four hours. He lectured for most of the time, an impressive feat, and he lectured fluently, though almost always from manuscripts. The density of wordplay, the homophonic associations Derrida always delighted in, sometimes made it seem like I'd walked in during the middle of an ongoing performance of some strange experimental novel. I picked it up in parts, finally succumbing by the third hour to the mere rustlings of language. I watched a raven-haired girl in the row ahead fill line after line of graph-paper notebooks in a neat minuscule hand, never stopping. She seemed to be able to take him down verbatim. Here was the sort of *parisienne* I'd fantasized about running me over on her bicycle: pale, petite, delicate, wearing a miniskirt and black stockings with braided stripes, and a soft-colored, lavender-scented blouse. I imagined her eating two bites of a goat cheese salad, accepting a date to see some Jim Jarmusch movie with a soft breathy *"Oui,"* exhaled from small, pert lips with that Parisian hiccough at the back of her throat; I imagined her bicycle, her lesbian affairs. I started to buy the same kind of orange-covered notebook she used, and once, after class, followed her to a café. She sat down near the front and I stayed outside, pretending to wait for someone else, smoking a series of cigarettes while I watched her through that perpetual screen, the Parisian *vitrine*. She drank an espresso, crossed and uncrossed her legs, looked up toward the door, and reviewed her notes.

In January, Saamer announced he was going to join the Bosnian mujahideen, still holding off the Serbs in Sarajevo, and disappeared for a few weeks. Again, I thought of Julien Sorel, who, just at the moment when he seems to have surmounted his provincial origins and climbed to the heights of Parisian aristocracy, just as he's about to marry the most desirable and head-strong woman in Paris, throws it all away in a kind of suicide that not even Stendhal seems to have fully understood when he wrote it. Something in Julien's character revolts against the very fairy tale he'd willed himself to live, and Stendhal let him go blow it all up, because—I guessed—self-destruction was as much part of life in the nineteenth century as now.

I was beginning to work on the seminar presentation I'd scheduled for March: on the biblical book of Jonah, and what Derrida said was its contribution to a Judeo-Christian rhetoric of hospitality, related to an ancient concept of "cities of refuge." A city of refuge was a place where, if you'd committed a crime by accident, manslaughter rather than murder, you could go live without fear of revenge from the family you'd wronged. I don't know what drove me to think about this idea so much that I offered to present on it, unassigned. I felt guilty of nothing except being young, fairly rich, and alive. Those weren't really things one was supposed to feel guilty for, but it wasn't something I couldn't not feel guilty about either.

I worked sporadically on the presentation as days became weeks, discovering that I neither knew enough Hebrew nor had enough understanding of the city of refuge to make a coherent point, or perhaps the only conclusion I had was one I was too frightened to make: that all our cities were now cities of refuge, that we were all guilty of harming people unintentionally, and we lived on only by divine sufferance.

My fantasies of accidental death returned. I put off a visit from my mother and, in a fit of impulsive responsibility, applied to American graduate schools in comparative literature, just as if pretending I had some grand plan all along could make it so. Saamer also came back after a few weeks. He'd got only as far as London, where Helen had followed him and pleaded with him. We resumed our old ways, although with a new, politicized edge. In late February, the neofascist National Front won the mayoralty of Vitrolles, a suburb of Marseille. The party was made up of angry veterans from France's lost colonial wars in Algeria and

Vietnam, Vichy sympathizers, a set of crazy reactionaries who wanted to restore the kingdom of Charlemagne to a state of non-existent Franco-Gaulish racial purity, former colonists who'd lost their power and property when France returned Algeria to the Algerians, but mostly unemployed white men, angry and bored. The newspapers I dutifully read daily in order to make myself feel more and more French were all alarmed. It was the first time the National Front had actually gained some executive power, and no one knew what they would do with it. Suddenly, Derrida's abstract inquiries into hospitality seemed more pertinent. Was France going to unlearn the lessons of its history, forget about Liberty, Equality, and Fraternity for all?

Saamer, Helen, and I joined the protest marches against the National Front that filled the streets from the Place de la République down to City Hall. I'd been reading Flaubert's *Sentimental Education* and had reached the part where Fréderic Moreau misses the revolution of 1848 because he's gone off to bed with a woman he doesn't really love. I was determined not to be like Fréderic Moreau. Allowing myself to be overtaken by events was a good, if oddly familiar feeling. I wanted to feel historical, to be carried along in the tide of the times. I decided I'd go to Vitrolles and write about what I found there. The most influential American journalist I knew in France was writing about Parisian department stores and bistros for Tina Brown's *New Yorker*. If he would not do it, I would.

The first week of March, I bought a ticket for Marseille on the high-speed train and headed south. There were rumors about French history books removed from libraries, Nazi-style torch-light marches, but I was disappointed by the silence I found, the apparent shame of the victors, who no longer even wanted to say anything racist that I could put into print. Maybe no one wanted to talk to a twenty-two-year-old kid without the official press credentials they demanded whenever I tried to enter a government building. *"Que les autres nous foutent la paix!"* was the only thing

they said to me, "Let other people leave us the fuck alone!" Those
other people could be Parisians, reporters, and, probably, the Arab
immigrants who were no longer even immigrants but second- or
third-generation citizens. Not only the ability to make your voice
heard comes with power, I realized. With power also comes the
ability to keep silent and keep secrets. The only people who'd
talk to me were the angry and disempowered Arab kids I met,
because they'd been able to speak honestly only among themselves. They were glad to have a random traveler and self-
appointed ambassador from the metropoles of Paris and New
York who would take a fleeting interest, transcribe their testimo-
nies, and then try to pass them off to American editors, most of
whom cared as much about goings-on in Vitrolles as most French
people did about the reelection, that same year, of a certain
governor of Texas. As it turned out, some of those kids could also
complain to wealthy Saudi fundamentalists who would teach
them to make bombs and fly airplanes.

I returned to Paris, after two days, to discover that I'd missed
the date of my presentation. It had been scheduled for the day of
my return from Vitrolles, not the following week, as I'd told myself. By some lights, I appeared to have made a decision: farewell
to the abstruse haunted musings of deconstruction and hello to
the rigors of serious investigative journalism. That was how life
was supposed to happen. But I hadn't made a decision, at least
not intentionally. It had been an accident, not as fatal as the ones
I'd imagined, but something silly and simple, like Saamer forgetting his keys. I believed in accidents, the slip of a needle, for instance. They were indicative of nothing more than the fragile
tensions in which our lives were held. As I saw it, I'd committed
nothing more than a "faux pas," a misstep; I'd got carried away
in the enthusiasm of the political moment and forgot myself in
an excess of solidarity with those who seemed to be in a more
precarious position than I was.

I rehearsed this case in my head before I decided to plead it before Derrida himself. When I showed up again at the office, there were no more books than the first time. It was always no more than a temporary space. He remembered our first meeting. Fortunately, he seemed to have forgotten that I was the person who'd stood up the seminar the week before. When I told him, he seemed confused rather than angry. There were usually two presenters and whoever was supposed to present with me had apparently taken advantage of my absence to speak for twice the normal length and so taken up the class. I told him about Vitrolles, and he seemed interested, at least enough so as not to be angry. He thought he could reschedule me for the following academic year, right at the beginning, in November. "You understand," he said, *"que voulez-vous?"* He shrugged like a Lower East Side grocer. *Que voulez-vous?* is a colloquial expression, a rhetorical question that signifies powerlessness and submission to a larger will, usually bureaucratic. Literally, it means "What do you want?"

Taken literally, it was a good question. And I didn't have an answer. What did I want, from him, from France? Why had it been necessary for me to go there at all? All that comes back to me, in belated response, is another scene in *The Red and the Black*: when Abbé Pirard, Julien Sorel's mentor at the seminary he's been forced to attend after his affair is discovered, tells him that he will not be a priest but a private secretary to the powerful Marquis de la Mole, in Paris, the grand capital of nineteenth-century desires. Overcome with gratitude at his liberation, Julien falls on his knees and tells the abbé, "I've found my father in you." It's an embarrassing moment of sentimentality for both characters, and Stendhal plays up their embarrassment. Julien knows the abbé will think he's being a hypocrite, and he's not sure whether he is. The abbé loves Julien's demonic energy but distrusts his own motives for helping him. It even seems like an embarrassing betrayal of the novel, which, like its hero, can never make up its mind whether the search for surrogate fathers is a flight from true freedom or a step on the way to liberty. I'd wanted Derrida to deliver me up to the freedom of my own mind, as though he could do it with a benediction, a wave of his hand. He did it instead with that shrug of his shoulders, and I hadn't realized it: "Truly they were in the father without knowing him."

I would not be back the following year, it turned out. Out of the blue, one afternoon, while I was working up my Vitrolles notes, I was interrupted by a phone call from the chair of Yale's Comparative Literature department, who was inviting me to enroll the following year with a full stipend. D called from Cambridge that same day to tell me he'd also been admitted, and, all at once, alone in the Parisian room that seemed so pregnant with accidental dangers, including, no doubt, some I hadn't even foreseen, I missed our nights spent together in search of that final, elusive meaning of literature. The idea that D and I, together, could rewind time and live once more sheltered by "the persistent critique of what we could not not inhabit" was too tempting to turn down.

Before I left, Saamer wanted me to come with him and Helen to Syria. We tried to figure out how to get past the U.S. State Department warnings against traveling there and the Syrian government's rumored ban on Jews.

"We'll drive you over the border from Lebanon in the trunk of a car," Saamer said. "I can get my father's diplomatic passport. They won't search it."

Helen laughed, "We will all eat Damascus ice cream!" She said it was like no other ice cream in the world, rose and pistachio flavors of a cream so rich it was rolled out in sheets and hung on hooks, without melting. I put them off, saying something about how I would try to get an appropriate visa the following year, after I'd started graduate school.

A few months after I went back to America, I called Helen, one evening, when, noticing a certain color in the sky, or a cloud, like a long winding sheet trailing from the east, I found myself overcome by a sudden feeling of desolation. Perhaps, I thought, I'd really loved her and should have done more to make it known. Her voice came across the Atlantic in a flat whisper when she told me Saamer had driven a car off the side of a mountain road, outside Beirut. There were three other people in the car. I never asked why she hadn't been there, or anything else about the accident, which it most certainly was, although also it wasn't.

It was easier for me to believe it was his fault, somehow, knowing him. Without wanting to torment Helen with questions over details she couldn't even know, I imagined how he'd pushed the accelerator just enough, whipping around a hairpin turn so as to have no chance once they hit the oil slick, or how the other car coming just as fast in the opposite direction, but on the inside lane, veered first and gave him no time to react. Or maybe it was an argument or a giddy joke among the passengers, among whom I could have very easily found myself. Still, it was the position, "on the edge," he'd wanted to be in; he'd courted it. He'd died in character, I told myself, which made me feel somewhat better. But what did it mean to die in character? Wasn't the whole meaning of *accident* something that happened to you precisely outside anything you'd chosen for yourself, and who could have enough faith in human mastery to believe that death, or the manner of it, was something we were allowed to choose? Did it make any sense at all, as much as I wanted to say it did, to feel that Saamer's death was more fortunate than my father's? And then, what about those other lives carried away in his fall?

7

I turned out not to be the only one in my family who thought that the way someone died revealed something about how they'd lived. While I had been away in Paris, and then in my first year of graduate school, my father's older sister, Anne, a prolific novelist and essayist, had been working on her thirteenth book, a memoir about her and my father's childhood, *1185 Park Avenue*, she'd called it, conjuring an era, as New Yorkers do, with the magic of real estate. I'd known my aunt was working on a book that involved my father, but I hadn't realized she'd written so quickly, or I'd failed to realize how much time had passed. She'd been hard at work, while, among other things, I'd been reading Freud's *Beyond the Pleasure Principle*, in which he argues that we each seek to die "after our own fashion," and our deeply ingrained unconscious habits make up what he terms a basic biological "death instinct" that leads us to choose how we put ourselves in harm's way without knowing that we're choosing to put ourselves in harm's way.

The few times I'd tried to imagine my aunt typing at her small desk in a corner off her kitchen, I'd felt this shadowy fear of becoming what a French literary theorist would call "the narrated." My father, my mother, and I were being changed into characters in someone else's drama. Against the meaning my

mother and I were trying to make from our own lives there would
be a counternarrative, always somewhere in print.

Then it had happened. An advance reader's copy of my aunt's
book had thumped through the mail slot of the brownstone building in Brooklyn where I shared an apartment. I'd ripped open
the envelope and hurled the thing on the kitchen counter, letting
it marinate as I considered drowning it in the toilet, or burning
it in Prospect Park, or letting it slip absentmindedly behind my
growing library of theory books and French novels where it
could remain unread. Yet I'd always been a reader, even when I
was nothing else, and so, before I was aware of having decided
anything, I'd taken up the bound galleys and started to read, not
stopping until the end.

There were books that had changed my life, usually in subtle
ways, like *The Ambassadors* or *To the Lighthouse*, books that allowed me to understand how other minds worked, how my own
mind might work, books that gave me a certain vocabulary for
emotions, or books that made me a safe spectator of situations I
would otherwise have been afraid of screwing up if I'd found
myself in them. A book about my family was not that kind of
book. The scenes exploded on my consciousness. They seemed
to require some immediate action, but I wasn't sure what I was
supposed to do, or what I was supposed to make of it.

What I'd found, at first, was a more novel-like version of the
fairy tale my father had told me about growing up on the most
boring street in the world. My father had said, as if it were a
truth as universally acknowledged as the law of gravity, that his
father had married for money, but guided by my aunt's fluid,
present-tense prose, which put the past before me as an eternally
ongoing scene rather than as distantly recollected facts, I finally
felt what that meant: the endless afternoons of two unhappy childhoods, the absent or—when present—rageful father, who'd passed
his name on to the son he wished he hadn't had by the woman he
was unhappy with. My aunt had discovered their father's long-

time mistress, a married woman, and discovered, too, that he'd fathered at least one child by her, leaving them all his own money as well as the portion he'd inherited from my grandmother, cutting both Anne and my father out of his will.

Anne filled the air with their mother's cigarette smoke, conjured her afternoon card games, her confessions of uncertainty, of impotence. In her story, the mother who my father said he'd missed every day tended him ambivalently or not at all, while she made a confidante of her daughter. Unpracticed with boys, she was afraid she'd be bad at dealing with them, and so my father was left to a hired governess. He grew up sickly, unathletic, intellectual, uninterested in the masculine worlds of business, of tennis at their country club, an anti-Semite's idea of a yid in a house determined to remain Jewish without ever looking too Jewish. He'd been sent home from school once for something unspeakably shameful that had resulted in an early course of preadolescent psychiatry. As a teenager, he became sincerely, devotedly religious, awkward or indifferent around girls; later, shedding religion without explaining it to my aunt, "as a snake might shed its skin," she wrote, he'd discovered music, opera, and the novels of Proust and Thomas Mann. His mother once set up a girl he seemed to like with another boy. "I had my reasons but I can't explain them to you," Anne remembered being told. All this, like a thin-spun thread through the book, led to an inevitable conclusion or half conclusion, the connection made clear in a lament against the sibling mistrust they never managed to overcome:

> He did not tell me he was sick until nearly a year and a half after he had full-blown AIDS pneumonia and then he swore me to deepest secrecy. Of course I considered the fact that I might still not have the full truth. If he did not, even then, tell me everything about his life and if his AIDS was in fact contracted in the more usual way I would have been heartbroken—heartbroken because he

would have lived so long bending beneath the deceptions
forged in other ignorant and cruel times.

I stumbled over these sentences. Why would anyone write such a
thing in a work of "nonfiction" memoir? I wondered. She was
outing him without outing him. There was a safety in that conditional, the subtlety of an otherwise superfluous "in fact." Was
Anne trying to avoid the truth of my father's obvious bad luck?
Or did she know more than she let on? I was reading the book in
what was basically a finished draft. It had been sent to me a few
weeks before it was due to be sent out to book reviewers and
magazines. Had she been trying to protect me until the last possible moment, or did I even matter to her at all?

Throughout my childhood, I'd heard how Anne was not
being spoken to by some family member or friend who'd taken
offense at something she'd written. Her first novel, *Digging Out*,
like many other first novels, was largely autobiographical: her
account of watching her mother's slow death from melanoma. It
was an angry book, verging on outright satire in more than a few
places. I also thought there was a lot of bravery in it. The nou-
veau riche and terminally anxious Park Avenue society my aunt
described held strict taboos against discussing death too openly,
death and, perhaps more important for my aunt, the wasted life
that had gone before it. Even when her novel was published, in
the nearly revolutionary year of 1967, various superstitions and
rumors still clung to cancer: people thought the disease might be
contagious, or was caused by psychological repression or deep
unhappiness instead of genetic triggers and long afternoons sun-
bathing with cigarettes. My aunt, too, was sometimes guilty of
letting melodramatic metaphor intrude on scientific truth, and
my father had once pointed out a sentence where she wrote of
"cancer cells crawling over the corpse . . ." as an example of how
unreliable she could be about matters of fact. Even if cells could
crawl, he'd said, these were as dead as the person.

My father had escaped unrepresented from that first novel and her subsequent ones as well. "My sister is an only child," he'd liked to complain, whenever anyone would ask him if her accounts of their family were true. Perhaps he ought to have taken it as a pale sign of her love for him, protecting him from whatever impulses led her to describe a character based on our infamous relative, Roy Cohn, like this: "Bernie's testicles, which had descended slowly and not completely, now in his early twenties seemed to have sunk back into the soft flesh of the lower stomach where, like unharvested grapes, they wrinkled."

Roy Cohn probably deserved that for helping Joseph McCarthy ruin the lives of hundreds of left-leaning innocents, for being a closeted gay man working near the top of a political party that had recently made homophobia a campaign platform. No, he deserved worse. But once it was my father's turn, I began to wonder how much Anne's avenging lash was within her control.

The way my father had explained it to me, he and Anne had seen their way through a normal sibling rivalry to occupy distinct positions in the world. Nothing was out of the ordinary, although it was clear he wouldn't trade places with her. She was the novelist, the purveyor of fictions and fantasies, a person of dubious value to humanity. He was the scientist who dwelled in facts on the ground and on the molecular level. He broke things down into discrete parts and patterns while she built castles in the air. It was normal, as he'd said. But for his accident, I imagined they'd still be circling each other in this uneasy but natural tension, the two cultures personified, masculine science, feminine arts, objective and subjective truth, eternally divided and eternally related, part of the predicament of our age. Instead, it had fallen to my aunt to have the last word.

I picked up the phone, about to call my mother, but stopped short of dialing. If she'd read the book, she probably would have called me already. If she hadn't, I didn't want to be the one to bring her the news. Exactly as we'd feared, my aunt was writing us into her version of the family script: my father was a failure, a casualty, not because of a mistake, but due to a hidden flaw in his character—not that he was gay but that he was too timid to admit it—and that made him unfit for the classic American story my aunt wanted to tell, a story in which each generation was supposed to be richer and freer than the next, from poverty to Park Avenue to, finally, happiness, the perfect or near-perfect union of the person you desired to be with the realities of your everyday existence. My aunt had succeeded in digging out and now posed as the elect looking back and down on the damned.

It was true that it had never occurred to me to doubt my father's version of events. I had nothing really to oppose to my aunt's suspicions except my own fragile and partial memories, and my maturing skepticism about neat literary truths. Her descriptions of my father did seem like secondhand borrowings from Freudian studies of homosexuality, back when psychiatrists believed it was a curable perversion or a lamentable condition, the outcome of family habits of child-rearing rather than a deeper biological imperative. My aunt had shown her readers a strong yet absent and spurning father, the coddling female who was not my unknown grandmother but my father's governess; there was my father's ambivalence about or lack of interest in his age's supposed manly pursuits and his turn to supposedly effeminate things such as music and literature. Even if these caricatures were sometimes true, just because many gays liked opera did not mean that all opera lovers were gay.

I'd said something like that last sentence to my aunt, when, after pacing up and down my apartment for a while, clutching the cordless, the Yankee game on the radio, I realized at last that I was going to have to call her. She suggested we talk about it in person at her place on Riverside Drive, in a tone I couldn't quite figure out. I was getting dragged back into it all again, and meeting at her apartment seemed like an added punishment.

I'd sworn to avoid the Upper West Side when I'd moved back to New York, both for the associations I dreaded encountering on each block and because of what I'd no longer find there. I'd become a stranger in what was turning into a contemporary American no-place: bank branches and Starbucks were sprouting up on every block of Broadway; chain bookstores had combined with rapidly rising rents to close down the bookstore where I'd worked. The movie theater where I'd watched *The Seven Samurai* with my ex-girlfriend and *Henry V* with my ex-father was also gone. A former neighbor I'd run into at a Brooklyn party told me that the movie producer who'd bought our home on Central Park West had refitted our music room as a fully equipped screening room, where opaque shades now lowered automatically to block the light. I supposed I ought to have welcomed the way these landmarks of my past were almost entirely erased. Instead, by some obscure mental law, their absence only made me all too aware of what was missing.

And so I showed up an hour early to meet my aunt, out of a fear of not showing up at all. I paced around her neighborhood for a while and settled at last in the sheltering cool of the Fireman's Memorial statue, a seated marble giantess in white robes overlooking the Riverside Park esplanade up near 100th Street. I sat smoking in the shadow of what some early-twentieth-century sculptor had intended to be an allegory of "duty" or "sacrifice," sorting through my thoughts, tracing lines with the toe of my boot in the dirt at the statue's base, not unlike the way I'd traced figures in my parents' carpets, wondering how my family's life might appear as a drawing: Would it be a graph of converging asymptotes, a labyrinth, a squiggly arabesque, or a sketch of a perpetually incomplete city, its landmarks ever shifting? Across the street, along the park esplanade, a kerchiefed old woman broke bread for pigeons, while on the bench next to hers, a bearded giant, wrapped in a duffle coat, shook his head from side to side, counting up cans and bottles he'd gathered in garbage bags at his feet. One leg of his pants was ripped from cuff to knee, as though slit by a knife.

For some reason, I was suddenly convinced that my aunt would have taken my remarks on the phone as a sign that I'd inherited the homophobic attitudes of those crueler times. She'd think I was trying to defend my father from the taint of gayness or bisexuality. She didn't know me that well. We'd barely spoken since I'd left college, and yet her judgments were ever quick, sometimes perceptive, sometimes wildly off the mark.

Would I really have to explain to her that gayness didn't horrify me at all? Would I have to remind her that I was a child of New York, the Athens of our age? That I'd grown up reading Mary Renault novels about Alexander the Great and his great love for Hephaestion, that one of my high school friends had lived in a townhouse on Twelfth Street, off West Fourth, in what was then New York City's signature gayborhood? On our way to the comic book stores off Washington Square, my friend and I had walked past mustached men in faux cowboy chaps, biker gear, and Nazi leather hanging out in front of a bar on Greenwich Avenue. As we got older, we'd looked in the windows of the lesbian Cubby Hole when we went out for underage beers at the Corner Bistro; we strode past transvestite prostitutes on our way to four a.m. breakfasts at Florent, and watched boisterous black drag divas leaving the Two Potato bar. These sights did not arouse anything stronger than amused curiosity, like street theater one was invited to observe without participating in. They provoked no reflections on Sodom—my friend, first-generation son of Indian anesthesiologists, had been notorious in our Dalton class for sighing "Ah, monotheism," during our ninth-grade English reading of the Bible, but he might as well have said, "Ah, sexuality!" We had no anxieties that the nerds we then were would be urged to take an active role in the pageant. They appeared no more ridiculous to us then than the rest of life.

But if I explained this to her, wouldn't she think I was too complacent, and maybe also covering up something? Did I know myself? From a hands-on perspective, my teenage sexual orientation had been neither homo nor hetero but auto, from which, I supposed, one could plausibly conclude that my favorite sexual organ must be the penis. Yet it was plain to me that I wasn't interested in anyone's penis but my own, and my imagination liked to pretend I was actually stroking the fine long breasts of some eagerly glimpsed girl, or that my hand had somehow found its way between her stockinged thighs, which rubbed together as she walked away from me down the block. Or maybe it wasn't the penis transformed, but my hand that became her tongue, or my hand became my tongue tasting her lower lip, or transformed into the elaborately manicured fingers of some Puerto Rican checkout girl that had earlier brushed my wrist while giving me change. Being before desire, in the way that Kafka's man stands before the law, I only imagined what was on the other side rather than how one got there.

By the time I read my aunt's memoir, I'd been propositioned by men on the street, my ass had been grabbed on the subway, penises had been flaunted at me in public restrooms; traveling, I'd been chatted up a few times in ways that ended more or less pleasantly with my refusals of invitations to stay over or come see something or other. I tended to take these interventions as compliments rather than assaults or invitations to consider whether I was somehow insufficiently showcasing my heterosexuality, whatever that meant.

"The full truth" my aunt wanted was a tempting and deceptive phrase. I found my grandfather's deathbed disinheritance of his children more immediately disturbing than the ghost of my father's possibly ambiguous sexuality. The barely known grandfather Anne described resembled the father I knew. Apparently, he had raged against "idiots" and "morons" in Truman's government in the tones my father had used when treating us to his own venomous outbursts against Reagan's "stupidity." I recognized, too, my grandfather's obsessions with privacy and secrecy, obsessions natural in a man with a secret life, anger natural in one constrained to play a role and eager for the play to end. Without realizing it, my aunt had revealed that my father had been, despite every effort, a different kind of good son to his own father, repeating the same estranged life in a different key. I worried that I, too, would have no choice but to repeat my father without knowing it.

Beneath the statue, the lines of my family diagram were becoming more and more of a maze, a tangle of loops and knots. My aunt's account and my father's account of their childhoods differed so greatly in intensity I could only think that the truth was either being stretched or suppressed. But which was it? My father had certainly been capable of lying, even lying cruelly. My aunt had unwittingly recorded just such a moment. During one of their last visits she'd reached for his glass of water, to take a sip, and he'd shouted out at her, "Don't drink that! Do you want to die?" In her admitted ignorance of microbiology, she took it as a sign of his concern for her, a family bond that persisted despite years of mistrust. But this was, I believed, sheer terrorizing. You can't get AIDS from drinking from the same glass as someone with the disease, at least I thought you couldn't, because I had often shared glasses with my father to show I wasn't afraid of him. I could well believe that, even a few months before his death, my father would have been capable of replaying a childhood practical joke on his sister—"cooties." She'd been right to distrust him, just as my mother and I had been right to trust him.

Yet had we been right to trust him? I wondered, losing patience and blotting the labyrinth with swipes of my boot. If my aunt was right, if my father really had been "bending beneath the deceptions forged in other ignorant and cruel times"—the double entendre in that phrase was already almost unforgivable, re-

gardless of whether she meant it—then my own existence was
like a prop, a decoy to throw off nosy people like Anne. Was this
why he'd been so ready to move from disapproval to disinheritance, once he'd realized he had no further use for me?

I shook off these looming doubts and began the brief climb
toward my aunt's apartment building at the top of the hill, wondering whether I'd be able to explain any of this, or whether she
even cared to know. Ever since I'd first met her, which wasn't
until I was six years old, at a Passover seder at our apartment,
she'd seemed a person to impress and be careful around. She and
my father had recently made up after a long quarrel about the
way she described Jews—or maybe it was her decision to celebrate Christmas for several years before she returned to the kind
of Reform Judaism my father made fun of. Something about the
circumstances of their breakup and reconciliation meant that I
was being drilled to ask the four questions in flawless Hebrew
and with more than usual urgency.

All I'd been told was that my aunt and her two youngest
children were coming for Passover, but Anne's memoir confirmed
my suspicion that some sort of family pride had been at stake.
According to her, my father had already been vaunting my lin-
guistic prowess over the phone, as though launching their rivalry
into the next generation. "The boy," she remembered him telling
her, "has a perfect accent."

Mostly I remembered my excitement at this sudden broaden-
ing of my world. I had new cousins. They were girls! They were
older, by four and six years. I let them lead me around. They put
me into a trance, "light as a feather, stiff as a board," convinced
me I'd actually levitated several inches. They'd been reading the
Brontë sisters recently and wanted to play Gondal. I was their
page. I announced their entrance to the dining room with a flourish and went off into closets where they sent me on quests for
some hidden and all-powerful object.

After the relative success of that Passover reunion, my father and Anne seemingly agreed to exchange us kids for periods of time, as Mughal and Bedouin royal families used to hostage out their children to keep the peace. So I would go to baseball games with my psychiatrist uncle, at least until I got too upset by having to sit through a nineteen-run annihilation of our beloved Yankees, and, as my father put it, "humiliated him" when I cried and begged my uncle to take us home before the game was over. I was a quitter. Meanwhile my cousin Katie came to my father for Hebrew lessons as she prepared for her bat mitzvah. She impressed him, and he told me, as I increasingly avoided my father when it was time to resume my own lessons, that she might be the family's true intellectual.

Shortly before or shortly after my father got his HIV test results, my parents went to Paris for a few weeks—to visit friends, they said. I stayed with my aunt in the brownstone where she lived then, Ninety-fifth Street on the far East Side, four long blocks and an entire neighborhood away from where she and my father had grown up. In addition to the cousins I knew, my aunt's daughter from her first marriage would drop by, and sometimes my uncle's two daughters from his first marriage. There were two spaniels and two or possibly three cats. The youngest cat kept me up nights, pouncing on my feet in the bed. Before I was dropped off, my father explained that if anything happened to him and my mother, a plane crash, for instance, which I worried about, my aunt had agreed to take care of me. I couldn't tell if I wanted this or not. When things got bad at home, when I was applying to colleges, I remembered this arrangement, and told my parents that I wanted to move out and live with Anne, in part because I knew it would hurt my father the most, but largely because I felt my parents really had vanished, as if in some plane crash or car crash, and also, impossible to deny, because my aunt's house really was a happier place.

From what I had seen, she and her second husband, a child psychoanalyst, loved each other deeply and with a near chivalrous

grace that called up images of classy old Hollywood couples like
Hepburn and Tracy, Bogie and Bergman. He called her "lady" in
a way that managed to evoke the most intimate affection with a
kind of decorous distance. At Thanksgiving, if she asked him to
open the wine while he was still in the kitchen baking bread, his
easy baritone would boom out, "Listen, lady, if you think the
world runs according to your wishes, you are sadly mistaken."
This was a kind of light irony my parents seemed incapable of,
for all my father's jokes. In the same way, it was unimaginable
that my parents would slow-step together on New Year's Eve, the
way I once watched my aunt and uncle dance to Cole Porter tunes.

By the time I finally pushed open the heavy iron doors and
the doorman announced my name over the intercom, I was convinced this was going to be my last visit to a fantasy home, a
different childhood from the one I'd actually had. Even if my
aunt turned out to be right about how my father was actually
infected, to know more than any of us, I felt wronged by having
been told in such an impersonal and indirect way. Clearly she'd
cared as little for me as my father claimed she'd cared for him.
I'd never really belonged there.

A strange surge of patriarchal pride bore me up: last of the
Roths, at least legally, on my way to defend my father's reputation, my mother's honor. Here, at last, was an active role for me
to play, a man's role. My aunt might have even approved of my
playing it, since sometimes the voice of crueler and more ignorant times spoke through her, too, despite her avowed feminism.
When I'd told her I was applying to graduate school to study
literature, she'd replied, "It would be nice if one of the men on
our side of the family was interested in making some money."

In this memorial and defiant mood, I studied the lobby's or-
nate ceilings and decorative moldings as I waited for the elevator
to take me up. Faux-medieval heraldry gilded the ceilings. Creatures held up shields with various devices, a bend sinister, three
fleurs-de-lis. They looked as much like seals as the sirens or

dragons they were intended to be copies of. The walls were lined with neoclassical motifs, nymphs and fauns dancing around pastoral urns. And yet here I was, too, in Arcadia. For moments like these I had been given my expensive education, to see the ghosts of Medicis and Borgias behind this mid-twentieth-century fantasy of Renaissance living, to know they'd played out their family scandals beneath more well-wrought versions of the same ceiling.

My aunt was probably expecting me, or perhaps even wanted me, to come out indignant. She'd played that scene many times already, with her cousins, her aunts, even my father. I could come to her as a censor, threatening lawsuits, although I was also sure that she had chosen those conditional sentences precisely to forestall any legal action. If I did that, I'd become the latest of the Roth and Philips men to try to shut her up, to put the woman in her place, to deny the possibility of "full truth." I would be the villain in an American story of anyone's right to speak and write freely. I didn't want a replay of this tired scene, but I wasn't sure what else to do as the elevator carried me up to the fourteenth floor, and I turned the doorbell to her apartment, designed like the key to a windup toy.

My aunt opened the door, her unruly and perfectly white curls surrounding her sun-weathered and kindly face with a fuzzy sort of halo. She, too, was part of the childhood I had to lose. She smiled at me in a way that seemed partly shy. She'd always had a warm, wide smile that could have been cultivated to put people at their ease, but also seemed completely unforced. She beamed naturally in a way that simultaneously sheltered and put me in my place, a younger member of the tribe who'd earned the elder's benevolence. It was also my father's smile, as I noticed only some years later when I looked at one of the few photographs of them side by side. Despite the beatific look, her tone was businesslike as she offered me coffee and ushered me into the dining room, which I was used to seeing prepared for large family gatherings: seders, Thanksgivings, her birthday parties.

I went over and sat down on a cushioned windowsill, and, while I waited for her to bring back the coffee, stared at the views downtown and east. What had once been a clear shot of the Empire State Building was now hidden by Broadway's newer, shoddily designed skyscrapers of faux brick and glass. No matter how well you did for yourself in Manhattan, there was always something to remind you that your existence was ever entwined with other people, that you were stacked up with them, that your neighbor peered into your living room just as you watched him go into the kitchen, late at night, and raid the refrigerator in his boxers.

Privacy was an illusion, or another expense in a city skilled at repackaging what had been common to one generation as the luxury of the next. My father had put almost everything he had into the Central Park West apartment so that only trees spied on us through the high living room windows. To live in New York, however, as my aunt understood it, was to live in public.

When we faced each other, hands around our coffee mugs, I waited for her to speak. "This was not the book I set out to write," she began, and for a second I thought she was preparing an apology. "I went to my publisher with an idea of writing about hero scientists, about my brother as a heroic scientist. People who give up their lives in the course of their research. That was what I thought I was going to write, a story out of *The Microbe Hunters*, that book my brother used to read to you." She went on, more defiantly, it seemed. "So I began to research that book. I talked to people. People who knew your father . . . They told me certain things and I was reminded of other things I'd forgotten, from our childhood. And the story I wanted to tell started to seem wrong. It wasn't the story of his life."

"But what is the story?" I asked.

"The story is in the book," she replied.

I realized I had only one question for her. What did she know? Who or what were her sources? I didn't want to sue her or protest, only to demand what she'd said she also wanted: "the full truth." And yet I couldn't ask if that full truth also included her decision to spice up her memoir with an unproven piece of gossip. Neither really would I have been able to ask whether she had shifted onto my father the responsibility for his HIV as a way of writing about her daughter from her first marriage, who'd contracted HIV in her late twenties, either through injecting heroin or from a boyfriend on heroin.

My cousin, in our family way, had written her own book about what it was like to be a single woman, trying to survive with HIV, but the stories I'd read made almost no mention of Anne, and I didn't know how they were getting along or how Anne felt about it. Was it possible that her message of forgiveness to my father for not having told her the full truth was really a plea for her still living daughter to trust her? If my father had his reasons to insist on absolute secrecy, what were her reasons for insisting on his exposure? Those questions stayed in my mind, unspoken. The book was there, a fact of its own. I had read it. Nothing else mattered, at that moment, except finding out what she knew.

She wouldn't tell me. Not at first. There were problems. She had promised to protect her source, she said. I laughed. I remembered how my father said that she was always holding out something to him only to snatch it away. "Like Lucy with the football," he'd said. I told her that it seemed only right that I, too, should know what she knew. She said she would ask. We left it there.

Then, the coffee cooling, unsipped, she began to ask me about myself, my plans. It was a way of urging me not to dwell in this past she found herself returning to again and again, at the same time that she'd brought me back into it. All the same, I felt judged, inadequate, as though she was expecting to read in me the same lineaments of failure and unhappiness she'd traced in my father. She wanted a further triumph. The sun shone painfully bright through the high windows, heating the room. I sweated and felt like a specimen on a slide fixed for her to examine. I had to admit that things were not exactly working out, that I could offer no tales of successful novels completed, of a brilliant academic career in the works.

I'd taken a leave of absence from graduate school and re- turned to New York, more uncertain than ever. When my aunt's manuscript found me, I'd been lying on my favorite spot on the old rug I'd trundled with me from one apartment to another, wondering why I'd fallen two months behind on my rent for no good reason. My friend from high school, the one I'd shared my secret with, lived a few blocks away but told me he didn't really want to talk to me until I agreed to admit that I was depressed and probably needed to find some other shrink, take medication, or at least quit smoking and start jogging again. I had good days and bad days, a futureless, empty and ongoing present. Naturally, I mentioned none of this.

When I left my aunt's, I was oddly relieved to have got off and got away so easily, as though I were somehow in the wrong. Yet I was flustered by my failure to gain anything of use or to have reached a conclusion. In the spring air along West End Avenue, I remembered another story my aunt had once told me: one of the bits of information she collected in passing and liked to relate impishly. There are men, she'd told me, who, one day, for whatever reason, just leave everything behind, their families, their identities. They drive out somewhere: California, New Mex- ico, or another country, and just think they can begin again, afresh, afresh, afresh.

I could see she'd been thinking of my grandfather, who hadn't had the courage to leave completely but kept a secret wish for freedom bottled up as he took my grandmother's money and used it as a down payment on his second family. I also thought she'd meant to send a message to me, to tell me that I, too, could, at any time, break completely, disown the past, exit the family script, and, by leaving, also reenact our family's flight from Old World to New. Immigration could become a perpetual state, an uncontrolled ancestral desire, wanderlust rising up in every generation. For whatever reason, though, I could not will myself to forget, to leave it alone or cut myself off.

"It's up to you," my cousin, the one my father had called our true intellectual, said to me over the phone, later that afternoon, "to find out the truth." "I am trying to find out the truth," I said, "that's why I asked your mother." But I didn't really want to find out the truth about my father so much as I wished to be told, to have it up or down, as though I were once again fourteen and waiting in the air-conditioning to find out the horrible thing I must have done to make my father have an important talk with me.

8

I knew I'd have to ask my mother. It was like a slowly spreading virus, this need for the so-called truth. I arranged to meet her for lunch at an Indian vegetarian restaurant on lower Lexington Avenue—close enough to the chamber music organization where she worked and also far enough away that we were unlikely to run into anyone she knew. I'd picked a public place because I dreaded a scene. I didn't know what I was about to hear, but I hoped that the muted maroon walls, the serenely hanging little discs of silver, and the Ganesh statues would at least impose an alien calm on both of us, that we could sit there as adults conducting a meeting. I forgot that the restaurant specialized in rice-flour crepes known as dosas, and that crepes had been my mother's signature breakfast dish, the centerpiece of a hundred quiet Sunday mornings.

My mother had not been sent a copy of *1185 Park Avenue*, she said, so I was put exactly in the go-between role I'd dreaded. I pulled out the galley and showed her the passage. She read it slowly, as the dosas arrived, sending up wafts of curried potato and coconut chutney. They remained untouched.

"Is there anything to this?" I asked, without mentioning that I'd already spoken to my aunt.

"Not as far as I know," my mother said.

"Do you believe it?"

I waited, impatiently broke pieces off the dosa's shell, crumbled them into the sauce, pushed at them with the spoon and watched them drift.

"Dad loved you, loved both of us . . ."

"That's not the point," I interrupted—the way she called him "Dad" already set me off, as though she thought I was still incapable of understanding that the man she married and my father were the same person. Why didn't she call him by his name, which is how she must have thought of him—or did she? Was he her father, too? That made it worse. And, really, why would my father's putative bisexuality have anything to do with whether he loved us? Besides, I had no idea what *love* as a verb meant anymore. To me the word appeared to try to do something to you rather than describe anything. To say "I love you" was to say something like "I family you." My father once told me that old 1950s sex-ed joke about "sex being a horrible nasty thing you do to someone you love." At that moment in the restaurant, I was more likely to think that "I love you" was a horrible, nasty thing you said to someone you had sex with.

"Do you think it's true?" I asked her again.

She looked up at me, behind her lightly tinted glasses, measuring out her words.

"You know as much as I know."

I wasn't sure whether I should be relieved or more anxious. Then she said she was ready to call our lawyer. I had a brief glimpse of a future spent in interminable lawsuits to establish the truth about a dead man's sex life. I suddenly felt much older than my mother. It was just a stupid book, I said soothingly. There were wrongs that could not be addressed by the legal system. All the same, this feeling of my sudden maturity, my worldliness, filled me with a quiet despair. As I walked my mother back to her office, I couldn't help a sense that she and I had once more missed a chance to talk about what it had meant for us to survive my father's illness. I had never been able to ask her whether she'd ever thought of leaving him, whether she regretted the years of nursing him, or whether she kept bringing up the father of an old school friend whose wife had just died of cancer because she'd been having an affair with him and she couldn't quite bring herself to tell me.

Not long after this, my aunt called to say she'd spoken with her source and he'd agreed to talk to me. She spoke the name of my father's closest friend, who also happened to have been his boss, the hospital's chief of hematology. Victor was the one who'd come the morning of my father's death to help my mother clean up, the one man apart from his doctors whom my father had chosen to trust first and last with every detail of his disease, the one man he'd really had no choice but to trust. My shock competed with Victor's confusion when he and I faced each other alone in his apartment near the Museum of Natural History. He was a bear of a man, proud of his stomach, proud of his bristling beard, and he clapped me to him in a hug with one meaty arm. He suggested we go out for dinner, as though the feeding of information had to come wrapped in something more immediately nourishing or, like certain medicines, not taken on an empty stomach.

Victor began speaking before we left. He said he'd made a strategic error. He'd told Anne two things he thought would keep her from writing any book about my father at all. The first thing he told her was that the probability of HIV infection from needle-stick infections in the lab was very small. This wasn't a heroin addict injecting himself directly in the vein with a serum containing a fair amount of other people's blood, this had been a slip, a brief puncture made with a needle that retained perhaps a trace amount of the virus. It was true, Victor admitted, that data on accidental laboratory infections did not come to light until 1984, after my father was infected and after scientists had developed a drug that, taken within twenty-four hours of exposure, reduced the risk of infection to almost nil. Victor also

acknowledged he hadn't witnessed the accident, as, in fact, no
one had.

The second thing Victor told me was an anecdote. One night
in the early 1980s, in Chicago, while he and my father were at a
hematology conference, Victor was relaxing in his hotel room
when my father called and asked him to come out for a drink.
Victor was tired and begged off. A few minutes later, the phone
rang again, my father calling back to tell Victor he should come.
He was at a gay bar, he said. It would be a new experience for
him. Victor said he'd joked with my father about how he ended
up there, and declined politely. He had to catch a flight the next
morning. That was it. He thought nothing more about it. The
invitation had been both unprecedented and never repeated.

Did Victor really think my aunt would not write about this?
I asked him. I'd never thought an adult capable of such naïve mis-
judgment of how someone was likely to act. He'd presented her
with a mystery. He'd presented me with a mystery. I'd fully entered
into the labyrinth of the "full truth." It was too late to go back.
He repeated that he'd made a mistake. I pressed him to tell me
more but he said this was all he knew and all he'd told my aunt. It
was remarkably little to go on, I thought, and was disappointed
that such a revelation could reveal nothing but more confusions.
The fog of mystery had lifted onto another mystery. He seemed
remorseful, anyway, so I let myself be taken out to dinner.

Victor had been like an uncle to me. A Chilean Jew whose
parents had fled Germany as he later fled Pinochet, he'd brought
a cosmopolitan flair to our life. He lived well and broadly, collected art, wrote poems in his native Spanish, one of which me-
morialized my father. He'd given it to me to translate a few years
before. I realized I hadn't followed through and could no longer
find the typed-out sheet I'd tucked into some file or folder in one
of the boxes of odds and ends that had started to accumulate
and follow me around from room to room, city to city.

Victor asked what I was up to, and I told him, with a bit

more honesty than I'd shown my aunt, that I was thinking about going back to graduate school but continued to want to write fiction. He asked me what I'd been writing, and I shrugged and said not very much, certainly not as much as I'd hoped.

"To be a writer," he said, "you must have no other choice. It's from within, an irresistible need. If you can do something else, do it. I write poetry now and then, for pleasure, but I'm a doctor. It's good to have a profession, to have money. I say this to my own children. When you're young everyone wants to be some kind of artist. But maybe you are just young?"

He paid the check, over my protests, and I promised not to tell my mother I'd spoken to him, or what he'd said.

It was then on the long ride back to Brooklyn, to the tune of the rattle and squeak of the old red IRT number 2 trains, that I began to plot my father's revenge, my redemption, my revenge, my father's redemption. A gay bar! That was it? I had been to gay bars, sometimes, for a quiet drink with friends who lived down-town. There were good ones in the West Village. It did not make me gay, although I could feel uncomfortable. But when did I not feel uncomfortable? And the low probability of the accidental needle-stick infection? It was low probability, not impossibility! I stuck to my intuition that there was something exceptional about us, even if exceptionally cursed. My father deserved better from his friend.

This was also the time when the lowest high school form of gossip, the sex scandal, had become the stuff of utmost political importance, "high crimes and misdemeanors." Bill Clinton re-ally turned out to have had a sort of sex with that woman, but, even before he had, people had been accusing him of far worse. Although he'd escaped the worst consequences of his affair, it was clear that whatever lingering promise remained of his presi-dency had been destroyed. "The Personal Is Political," that slo-gan we'd learned in my college years, so important in bringing attention to the ravages of AIDS, so useful to the cause of women's rights, had become the banner of an inquisitorial right wing bent on total power. The new media, which so many of my high school and college acquaintances were rushing to join, were like my aunt's book: they'd supplanted verifiable truth with rumor, Enlightenment science with gossip. There were no more peccadilloes, only deadly sins. My vengeance, which would be a book, of course, would not only be a blow in defense of my cursed father but in the service of literature, of truth, of benefit to my fellow Americans. Fired with this newfound sense of purpose—I would prove everyone wrong—I phoned my aunt the next morning to tell her I'd spoken to Victor.

"It's nothing," I said to her, "circumstantial evidence, that story about the gay bar." And then my carefully meditated parting shot, so obscure she wasn't even supposed to know what I was saying, not at first: "I'm not against literature," I told her, because I knew she'd think I was, "but I wish you'd written something more like Henry James, like 'The Beast in the Jungle.' " I explained, "You know that story where the skeleton wasn't in the closet, the skeleton was the idea of a closet. Maybe my father only fantasized about sleeping with other men and didn't actually do it. That's why he called Victor from the bar. He was nervous. Then he got sick by bad luck. Like being punished for wishing for something. We think that what happens to us are the most important moments in our life, but what if the most important events are the ones that don't happen?"

There was a little silence on the other end (had my blow struck?), then she spoke, "He's your father as well as my brother and one day you'll tell the story in your own way, if you want to."

I told her I was planning on it.

9

A few weeks later, I drove up to New Haven to look for an apartment and arrange my return to Yale for the fall semester. The leave of absence I'd taken after my first year of graduate school now seemed like a purely irrational act: an obedience to the familiar feeling of disappointment and displacement I'd had at Oberlin, in Paris, and, even before, when my parents kept switching me out of secondary schools and summer camps. I understood that my first response to arriving at any place would be an immediate wish to leave, and that I'd become extremely gifted in plotting escapes, and even escapes from my escapes. Though determined to prove my aunt wrong, I didn't feel ready to write a book that had no form or shape in my mind except that of an antimemoir. I needed, like James Joyce, "silence, exile, and cunning," or just someplace that was going to pay me to read and not care if I did some writing on the side, which Yale was still prepared to do.

On my way up, I missed the exit for the Cross County Parkway and found myself driving north instead of east, passing Hastings-on-Hudson, where my father was buried. I made a turn I somehow remembered from when my mother and I had last been there, at the gravestone unveiling, five years before. The cemetery gates were open, but there was no one at the country cottage–style lodge. I parked at the base of the steep, terraced slope and began to follow a winding trail past the gaudy art-deco tombs of the first tier, Irving Berlin and the Guggenheims in their heavy marble funereal pomp. Impatient to ascend, I left the trail and began a straight charge through the graves, certain I knew where my father was buried, near the very top of the slope.

At the top, I wandered left instead of right, or right instead of left, looking for the bent-trunked cherry tree under which I was certain I'd find him. The Westchester Hills Cemetery turned out to be two, maybe three, different cemeteries: Reform Jewish on one side, and, on the slope's other half, Catholic and Greek Orthodox, an American dream of the tolerant afterlife, not so different from the city where these countless bodies had once lived. No visible border separated them, only a long, curving, tree-lined alley, which I must have crossed at some point, because I was wandering among Celtic and Byzantine crosses and statues of angels. I stopped at a marble bench with the word *Eros* written in both Greek and Roman script. I looked at it for minutes, not understanding what this pagan tribute was doing either in a Jewish or Christian place of rest.

Only when I sat down on Eros and faced the graves did I realize they were a family, a large one by the number of names inscribed along the bench's curving base. I wondered if I shouldn't take it as a sign; was it love triumphing over death? "Dad loved you, loved both of us?" Or death and family reaching out to claim even Eros, builder of cities. I couldn't decide, but they cheered me, the Eroses or the Erotoi, whoever they were.

I trudged back down the slope to the lodge, and found the caretaker, maybe the same man who'd buried my father with the bulldozer, promoted now. We located my father on the numbered map of plots, and I set off again. By the time I arrived, sweating in the haze of the humid afternoon, at the tree that was not a cherry tree, the river hidden behind a rustling summer wall of green and the peaking gables of a new, middle-class, mock-Tudor housing development, it was difficult not to feel that I'd gone looking for him in the wrong place. When he picked out the plot, my father had joked that he was moving, at last, to the suburbs. I thought about his body under the soil: bones by then, eight years on. There he lay, close enough to my mother and me to make us feel guilty for not visiting, far enough away to ask to be forgotten, a Jew among Jews, even though he hadn't allowed us to say Kaddish. God, who didn't exist, was not merciful, worth neither extolling nor sanctifying.

The flat headstone was almost completely covered over with grass and weeds. I cleared it to look once more at the inscription we'd chosen: "Eugene F. Roth, Jr., 1939–1993. Husband, Father, Scientist." The epitaph listed his social roles but could not encompass his life. It wasn't much and it left out a great deal. As a memorial it falsified him, it seemed, as much as my aunt's book had done. My father's epitaph could have read "Lover of Mozart, Rossini, and Cimarosa," as Stendhal's did, or "Lover of Proust, Mann, and Shakespeare," for he loved them, too, and with what seemed a far purer pleasure than he loved his research on malaria vaccines, or me, or my mother. Maybe we should have just had the courage to write "Eros."

Down again in the car, retracing my way back to the missed turn, I began to think again of those writers and their novels, among the pages of which my father might have felt most fully alive. If I were to look for him, to salvage his reputation from my aunt's portrait of the enfeebled, timid homosexual manqué, the kid brother, it would be among them, his true secret and unfulfilled loves. I tried to remember the stories and novels he'd put in my path when I was teenager and he was dying. A list came to mind, then: *The Metamorphosis*, *Tonio Kröger*, *The Red and the Black*, *Oblomov*, *The Way of All Flesh*, *Fathers and Sons*. I used to think these stories were the sort of stories any "normal," loving, well-educated, and emotionally reticent father might give his son to read. They were supposed to let me understand my own untidy adolescent feelings about families and the apparently cruel ways of the world.

The novels and stories I recalled all belonged, in more or less clichéd ways, to a long European period from 1842 to 1920 that tracked the rise of the liberal, upper middle classes to the brink of their destruction. They were mostly tales of acculturation or development—*Bildungsromane*—even as they represented a late and often self-critical stage of this genre. Their self-conscious belatedness, in most cases, seemed to reflect the situation I found myself in at the end of the twentieth century. Mine was the first generation in a while that seemed to regard replicating its parents' achievements, or at least their income levels, as a goal both desirable and worthy. Not for the first time, prominent intellectuals had declared history to be at an end. There seemed nowhere to go but sideways, or around in circles, like Gregor Samsa, the man-roach, crawling up and down the walls of the bedroom where he was confined.

For the first time, I began to wonder if I'd misread my father's intentions when he'd handed these books to me, or brought them up, often in response to my halting attempts to tell him an original thought I'd had. Perhaps, for all the moments of resonance with my own life that I'd recognized on the few occasions that I'd followed my father's recommendations and read about these ambivalent and doomed young men, it was my father's life all along that he was trying to pass on to me through these encrypted transmissions of what it felt like to be him. Read properly and carefully, these books would provide a far stronger and clearer portrait of my father than the one in my aunt's book.

Had someone else, my more critical cousin, for instance, been sitting next to me as I followed my father's preferred route to New Haven, along the loops, curves, and deer crossings of the Merritt Parkway instead of the straight path of I-95, she might have wondered if I was making a mistake. "Don't you know," she'd say, "Western literature is about so much more than You or Him? You have your own memories, don't you? Why must you mix everything up like this? If you really want to know whether your father cheated on your mother with men, if he had a steady lover or just went looking for the most dangerous kind of random encounter, why not launch your own investigation? Believe your mom, if you want, but how do you know Victor's told you everything? Call him back. Call my mom's friend, the one who went to college with your dad. You might find something out."

But I was alone, and what I wanted anyway was something greater than mere factual truth. I wanted my father, the man, not just the AIDS patient I remembered. I wanted to know, too, how much of who he was before and even after illness seized him had been passed on to me, whether there was any escape from family unhappiness, our curse, that did not require me to seal myself off from the past entirely, to floor the accelerator and keep going beyond New Haven, toward an entirely new life, somewhere out there in the open. Someone else, driven by some greater immediate necessity, the lack of money, for instance, might have been able to do this, to will forgetting. No more backward glances. But I could not. I wanted to be one of those people on whom nothing is lost—or one of those people for whom loss is everything.

10

The Department of Comparative Literature held its holiday party in early December, before most everyone fled the biting New Haven winter for at least a few weeks. In our damp and cigarette-scented clothes, my fellow graduate students and I piled into a narrow elevator, incongruous dynamo among the neo-Gothic archways and gargoyles, and rode up to the department's private library on the eighth floor of an old campus tower. I often went there outside official hours, hoping to find myself alone. In daylight, I could look out from all sides at New Haven's urban desolation, hoping for a glimpse of sea beyond the concrete band of I-95 and the Brutalist high-rise parking garages; by night I watched the room's warm reflected glow in the heavy glazing of an earlier modern age.

A mute literalization of the ivory tower, the library seemed set up to inspire lofty and abstract thoughts. I remembered how the department's secretary, a tough remainder of New Haven's vanished working classes, had handed me my key to the place with a sardonic flourish. Inevitably, the place reminded me of the secret castle room where, at the end of the original bildungsroman, Goethe's Wilhelm concludes his apprenticeship and is allowed access to the scrolls and books of the secret society of educators who have been his clandestine guides throughout his young life.

Whatever its original high intentions, the library was in decline when I got there. The books, donations from retiring or dead professors, were shelved haphazardly; the most recent journal on the recent-journal stand dated several years before my arrival. A second study room, off the main one, resembled our old Central Park West apartment as my mother and I were moving out of it; books stacked too high in open boxes had toppled and fanned out over the floor. An open ledger, placed on a lectern near the door, shyly asked people to sign out the books they took from this archive of neglected knowledge. Undergraduates or graduate students themselves were rumored to make out on the cracked leather couches, and a cautionary tale of academic poverty made the rounds about the former PhD who'd squatted in the library while commuting to part-time teaching jobs at three nearby community colleges.

At the party, though, all signs of decay had been momentarily swept away. A fire crackled in the usually dormant fireplace. A buffet spread of cheeses and sweets covered the wooden seminar tables. The department's various factions mingled uneasily in brief truce from their ferocious competition for dwindling prestige, funds, and student followers: the old deconstructionists greeted the last of the even older philologists, and together they ignored the new historicists. The junior professors either chatted with their students and showed off their newborns or took the chance to laugh at the jokes of those who'd decide their tenure cases.

I drifted into a little flock of gossiping graduate students. They discussed which professors had worked or still worked for the CIA, who was having an affair or had married for the third time, who was secretly or not-so-secretly gay, who was an alcoholic, and who lived as a shut-in. Never before had I known or half known so much about people I'd barely met or only spoken to in passing. There was such an abundance of stories that it made it hard to form my own sense of these people, what they stood for, how far their kindness or interest in me might actually extend. Behind all the gossip, I thought I detected something more than prurience: we wanted to understand our professors, with their varying brilliance and their rather ordinary ethical challenges, as reflections of what our potential future selves might be like, and sometimes we recoiled from those selves with a sharp disgust, a preemptive disappointment in the lives we hadn't yet led. Of course it was possible that some of the chief tale-tellers, the older sixth- and seventh-year graduate students, already felt themselves to be avatars of a new system, a new age of university life in which there would be no more affairs, no more uncomfortable compromises between power and principle that were smoothed over by the two or three or four drinks at each university function, topped off by the nightcaps in the empty suburban house with a view of the man-made lake or the blasted limestone cliffs of New Haven's better neighborhoods. For these students, our elders were simultaneously victims and beneficiaries of an old, semifeudal order of academic life, a less enlightened and crueler age now being replaced. Everything was going to be organized differently, they said, whether mandated by the management types in the administration or self-organized by a union of students and faculty.

I hadn't understood that I was being asked to choose a side in these ongoing struggles when I'd decided to return to the shelter of the academy. It was undeniable, however, as the end of the semester approached, that I'd been swayed away from the mystery of my father's life. "Why do you want to get into that *Oidipous Tyrannos* shit?" my old friend D said, when I told him about my aunt's memoir and my projected riposte. I couldn't help but agree. Family introspection was starting to seem a tiring and unrewarding profession, even though my aunt had made a living out of it. There was so much more that I wasn't related to: other languages to learn, books that neither my father nor my aunt had read, the coming student revolution.

Our department chair had ordered Australian Shiraz in surprising quantity. As the party thinned out and the older faculty
left, the bar became self-serve. I wandered over to the fireplace
with a couple of pilfered bottles and started pouring rounds for
a band of British graduate students. Whether it was the advanced degrees many of them already had from Oxford or Cambridge, or an academic culture that valued the ability to argue on
one's feet—one of them told me she used to play a game in which
you had to speak on a randomly drawn subject for five minutes
without stopping or saying "um"—they all seemed to project
a polished suavity and astonishing articulateness that actually
seemed to increase in proportion to the amount of alcohol they
consumed. I admired them for this, imitated them when I could.
Mostly this meant that I got drunk fairly often, not in a rowdy,
puking way, but not in an improved, articulate way either.

I did discover that I could maintain a certain self-control past
a point when quite a few others just gave up and enjoyed whatever part of themselves their drinking brought to the surface.
This made me a good straight man or sometimes just a dogged
listener, which was what happened when a slender, dark-haired
member of the British brigade pronounced himself enthused to
have a met "a genuine New York Jewish intellectual, and you even
look like Woody Allen," before pulling up and suddenly asking
me whether I could explain what he called this American obses-
sion with narrative. I wasn't sure what he meant by this cryptic
generalization about narrative, never mind about the Jews, and
told him so.

"Well, here at Yale"—he drawled the name—"there's a course
called 'Narrative and the Law,' taught in the literature department, and another one called 'The Law of the Narrative,' taught
by a psychoanalyst in the French literature department, and
then there's 'Narratives of the Dispossessed' and 'Intentional
Communities and Narratives of Colonial Repossession,' and
that's only this semester." He waved his free hand as if conducting

an unheard melody and tilted his head back, fixing a point on the ceiling. "It does seem like something people go on about here: Human beings are no longer just Aristotle's imitating animal but we're supposed to be the animal that plots everything. Our identities are supposed to have something to do with the stories we make up about ourselves or the stories we accept to have imposed on us. And our identities are supposed to be identical with who we are."

"And there's something wrong with this?" I asked.

"Well, it's not true, is it? I mean in every case. Here we are getting sloshed, but I can't tell you how that fits into the story of my life. I like a drink, and so do lots of people, but that doesn't mean that we all identify at every single moment as drinkers or oenophiles, and from the way you kept looking around after you picked up those bottles, I bet it's the first time you've raided an untended bar. And I doubt you did it 'cause your mum weaned you too soon. I bet most people don't even think of their lives as 'plotted,' in any meaningful way."

The melody picked up again and his hand moved, palm upward, as if summoning another instrument to play. "You ask them to tell you the story of their lives and they'll give you some heap of disconnected events: born here, parents split up, went to school, got a job, got laid off, moved to another place, got another job, married another woman, got sick, got well, hung around an inkwell. That's most people's lives, right, and it's a pretty boring story, although I guess it is a story. But suppose you ask them, 'What's the most meaningful thing that ever happened to you, or just your moment of greatest happiness?' and let's assume they're being honest, and you don't frighten them by telling them you're doing a survey on 'narrative self-conceptions' for university, they might choose something entirely out of keeping with what looks like their actual 'narrative' or story, like a trip to the seaside when they were young, even though they've never seen the sea since."

Before I could interrupt, he was off again, as if seeing the ob-
jection I was about to make before I made it. "You might say, oh,
he was really meant to be a sailor, or a fisherman, but he missed
his chance, and now he's in the glassworks, but that's also misleading, because maybe the great thing about being by the sea
was that it was simply outside anything else, contentless, it was
thrillingly unconnected."

In the pause, as he raised his glass, I wondered what to call
these people.

"Episodics," he replied, warming to his argument. "We can
divide people into two kinds, those who feel that their lives are
structured like a narrative, because I'm sure there are some people
like that, maybe at Yale, or in government, and those who feel
that life is a series of disconnected moments, transient and shifting desires: that, say, the fact that I played piano at age ten and
got really into Manchester club music at seventeen have little to
do with each other, and nothing at all to do with my mother once
closing the piano lid on my hands while I was practicing."

"But what about character?"

"But character is nineteenth-century fiction. I don't go
around asking myself whether going to this party is in character,
or having this conversation. I can have a party episode, a drinking
episode, followed by a study episode, a romantic episode, a professional episode—though one hopes that doesn't last too long.
It's situational: morality, ethics, character, identity."

In the red-wine haze of the evening, this argument sounded
convincing, at least as a description of my present circumstances.
How many times had I told myself that what I'd experienced at
the Dalton School, or during my fugal runs through Riverside
Park, were things that had happened to another person, a person
from whom I felt cut off, not because I was currently inhabiting
a false self that had been layered over the true one, but because
those earlier selves had dead-ended, were, in a sense, no longer
alive. They shared a body with me, true, but in the same way that

the corporate body of the Comparative Literature department contained multiple graduate students, some of whom, it had been made clear to us, would also dead-end and be released to become separate selves elsewhere.

Shortly after the party, with two unfinished papers hanging over my head, I traveled to Morocco with D. Fed up with all the millennial hype, we'd come up with the idea of going somewhere that wasn't even on the occidental calendar, changing time to suit ourselves. D's physique had filled out a bit since college. Thanks to a new hormone therapy that made up for his destroyed thyroid, he'd been able to start exercising. At twenty-six, he looked like the sinewy nineteen-year-old he hadn't had the chance to be. Along with us went Marie, recent ex-girlfriend of D's roommate Carl. It was supposed to be four of us, originally, but Carl and Marie broke up just before the trip, and Marie proclaimed she was still going, no matter what. So Carl changed his ticket to visit Berlin, and I found myself walking the streets of the modern quarter of Fez, one evening, while D and Marie remained at the hotel—perhaps the first time they slept together, or perhaps it had already happened before we left.

I settled on a café near the meeting of the old and new cities and sat among rows and rows of men who sipped tea and smoked, alone or with friends. A waiter set down a mint tea, without my needing to ask, and I took out the secondhand copy of André Gide's *L'Immoraliste* I'd been planning to start once we reached Tangier and the end of our journey. I'd chosen it more or less haphazardly, without knowing more than that it was partially set in Morocco. I might have been embarrassed that I'd never read Gide, as much as I claimed French literature as one of my specialities. I had a vague prejudice that he seemed too "classical," a more deliberately artful and therefore lesser Proust. I was unaware that the novel is the story of a young, married Frenchman's ambiguous acknowledgment of his attraction to adolescent boys. Nor did I know how the novel half embraces and half criticizes that choice, vacillating between a sense that nature itself might be not just amoral but actually immoral, sinful, and an ironic condemnation of any human order that could make love into an evil.

I started to dig in to Gide's novel and almost immediately fell into a different kind of irony, one of those vulgar everyday ones, bordering on the complete cliché, so obvious that it could only happen in reality, the novel perhaps having nothing to do with it, or the presence of the novel itself somehow inoculated me against acting out the cliché I was already half becoming. A guy, perhaps my age or younger, with the lithe muscles of a soccer player and the coppery black hair, high cheekbones, and green-blue eyes typical of the Berbers of the Atlas Mountains, slid into the squeaky, rusty chair next to mine and offered me a Marlboro. All sorts of people approached me in Morocco: selling things, offering themselves as guides, wanting to speak English, begging. I'd got used to it without liking it. But this boy's approach felt different. There was no immediate offer of service. We were just hanging out in the café. He spoke to me in French and Spanish. Just as I'd been taken for a Moroccan when I walked with Saamer in France, so, in Morocco, I was often mistaken for a French person, which I thought safer than being taken for a Woody Allen lookalike.

As we sipped our tea, I learned he'd been back and forth to Spain, like many Moroccan young men, working illegally; perhaps he'd been deported, and returned to wander his native streets, unemployed. We made the usual polite talk about the beauties of the city, of the country; he smiled at me and asked what I wanted. What did he mean, I asked. "Let's go for a walk," he suggested. I agreed. The winter air in the foothills of the Atlas Mountains had a crisp applelike cool, and I wanted to see more of the city after dark. After a block he linked his arm with mine and said, "Let's go somewhere, I'll fuck you in the ass, it will be beautiful." Where would we go, I asked. "I have a cousin," he said. I told him I didn't really want that. "Oh, I get it, you like it with girls. Me, too, sometimes. There is this place. Not too expensive. We go there. We get a girl. We take turns. Yes?" I suggested we keep walking for now. "But what do you want?" he asked again. I wanted to walk, I said. I tried to get him to talk about the politics of Berber nationalism, which he seemed about as keen to discuss as I was to visit a brothel with a complete stranger. It was a complicated country, Morocco. You could get everything you wanted except a frank exchange of views. At the next intersection, we said goodbye and he shook his head at me. "It would have been beautiful."

D was not in our room when I got back. Lounging on my bed, I tried to imagine what the strange boy might have felt like, the smooth pectorals of his bared chest, the coarseness of his coppery black hair under my fondling hand, the wild animal gleam of those green eyes, the jaw like some carnivorous animal's aroused at the thought of a feed. When had I seen or even pictured to myself another man's penis in full flagrant erection? Did I regret the opportunity missed, the untaken chance? The slightest slip in my resistance and I might have gone all the way toward realizing what had only been a theory about my father's other life, as if the rumor in my aunt's book had really been a prophecy intended for me. When is it an episode, when is it a narrative, and when is it just a repetition? I wondered, drifting off. Would it have been André Gide's fault? If I had multiple lives instead of the one and only, I would have gone through with the experiment. As things were, I simply felt too susceptible to influences, a creature spun out of other people's stories and wishes.

I returned to New Haven determined, once more, among political meetings, drinking sessions, and seminars, to resume my investigations. Haltingly, fearfully, at last, I began to read the books I'd chosen to search for my real father, the one I knew and the one who'd been hidden from me, whom I'd ignored. Sometimes I imagined I could see his face composing itself out of the various typefaces, shifting and changing expression with each paragraph, each chapter.

Sometimes the face blurred so that I could no longer be sure if it was my father's or my own, as had happened when I found his old passport in a box of his books I'd moved from my mother's new apartment. I'd opened it and there, gazing purposefully into the camera through slightly tinted glasses, was a young face, a wide mouth with lips curled slightly upward in a sardonic smile, as though mocking the bureaucrats for not giving him time to shave before the picture was snapped. His cheeks were still firm, with none of the excess weight they'd put on in four years and without the skeletal sallowness they'd acquire in another twenty-five. I checked the date of issue, 1964, two years after his mother's death. He was twenty-five, as was I when I looked at it. The twenty-five-year-old man in the photo was unknown to me, yet his face was mine or mine his. It was all getting mixed up.

Beginning to read my father's books created a similar kind of double exposure or superimposition of lives: my life and my father's life were on top of the lives of the characters and the authors. The stories I'd chosen were tales my father had passed on to me at an age when I assumed every character had something to tell me about myself. We first become ourselves by becoming someone else. Nearly everyone has this adolescent tendency to identify with literary characters, even when we should know better. My father had certainly never taken any pains to insist on the equally important work of differentiating myself from the people I read about. Thomas Mann's 1903 novella, *Tonio Kröger*, for instance, he'd begun reading to me one day when I was eleven years old.

I'd been taken out of the French school, which was supposedly on the brink of financial ruin, and found myself boarding a diesel-choked Liberty Lines bus with my violin, my French school-boy satchel worn across one shoulder, on my way to the more monied Riverdale School in the Bronx. My bag was very popular that year, with girls. "Are you a girl?" I heard at least once a day. "Why do you have that girly bag?" It was a boyish blue, I thought, but it didn't matter. Nothing mattered except that *girl* stuck to me. Innocently, someone might ask to see the bag, and, at the end of the ride, I'd be left to search for it among the far-back seats, pushing my way against the current of students filing off the bus, getting a shove or kick for my efforts. My glasses, too, sometimes were snatched. "He's blind, he's blind!" As soon as I got home, I ran into the living room, hid under the piano, pounding the floor, face streaked with tears of frustrated vengeance. I ditched the shoulder bag, got my hair cut, and clamored for contact lenses.

Around this time, my father had beckoned me onto the couch, and begun reading about a boy with a funny-sounding, mixed Italo-German name, a mother who played the piano beautifully, and a father "with thoughtful blue eyes," from an old merchant family. The boy waits in the rain outside the school gates for his best friend, Hans Hansen, who'd promised to walk with him and discuss Schiller's plays, but breaks his promise to run off with more popular boys and talk horseback riding and gymnastics, boys who belong to the race of "the tall and fair." Heartbroken as Tonio is, he understands that he is a creature apart, he will be a lover of music, of literature, and of athletic boys. He will not change and neither will they.

So much did I take this story to be about me that I acted it out, in my own way. One morning, almost at the end of the school year, the fire bells went off and we all poured outside, with the usual relief of children let out of school unexpectedly. As we lined up in our designated areas and waited, rumors coursed through the crowd of students. Someone's brother in the high school said that the fire drill was not a drill. A bomb threat was mentioned. Maybe we'd get the whole day off. The prospect was almost unbelievable, and then I remembered my violin; I'd left it inside the building. I needed to go back for it. I had to save it— the instrument had belonged to my grandmother, and I thought it was the most beautiful thing I'd ever owned. I told a boy I ought not to have trusted that I was going to sneak back in and get it. Caught, I was dragged back to the line, kicking and pleading, while my schoolmates jeered and laughed at the phrase I'd hear thrown back at me over and over for the few remaining weeks of my time at Riverdale, before my parents finally relented and switched me out, "Don't you understand? I need my violin. I am an artist."

In the context of its second coming, amid the Hanseatic gabled roofs of New Haven's graduate student ghetto, *Tonio Kröger* appeared more independent and remote, a creation of its own history and times. I learned that Thomas Mann thought of the novella as a lightly fictionalized version of his own childhood, and a reply to his earlier novel *Buddenbrooks*, about a rich merchant family that descends to decadence, bankruptcy, laziness, and "the artistic temperament," in three short generations. Instead of melodramatic decline, Tonio Kröger appears in the second part of the novella as a successful writer, yet, crucially, he regards himself as a diseased person, his artistic talents a curse, like inherited syphilis.

The necessary, fated unhealthiness and unhappiness of artistic consciousness was the sort of late-nineteenth-century convention that Mann picked up, played with, and yet had a remarkable fidelity to. I seemed to have absorbed it, unconsciously, by the slightest exposure, a distant beam from a dead star. Poolside, at my aunt's country house in Amagansett, one weekend when I was seventeen, while we watched my uncle at his early morning laps, she'd tried explaining to me that this idea of the artist as alienated and at odds with both himself and the world was an anachronism. She told me she'd been furious with my father for reading me that opening section of *Tonio Kröger* when I was, as she said, only a child. There was no reason that writers couldn't be as well adjusted and content as the bankers and lawyers they might write about, if not even happier. Her remarks at the time astonished me. Could one really have both happiness and art? It seemed dishonest, or at least unfair, to unhappy people like me and my father. If we had to share literature and the pursuit of truth with a bunch of well-adjusted people, we'd be left with nothing truly our own except our sense of failure. I'd started to love my aunt's swimming pool, the feel of the ocean when you stepped off the Hampton Jitney, the peace of money, but if I had to choose I knew I'd be faithful to my father's particular tribe.

Even though I didn't want to believe her, because her promise was so tempting, I also had to acknowledge a certain justice in what she said. My first acquaintance with *Tonio Kröger* really established "the artist" as an existential category of utmost importance in my life. I didn't need to be a loser, nerd, or freak; my particular unhappiness could be explained by a more dignified name. And so I'd adopted this word to describe myself before it was even clear whether I had any particular talents.

In my rereading, I began to wonder if my father hadn't deliberately confused Mann's metaphor of the artist as a diseased person with his own life as an actually diseased person, and whether I hadn't missed the point of his reading completely. Perhaps, to my father, I was cast more in the role of Hans Hansen than the titular character whose name seemed like my own. This was the problem with literary identification: there were no rules for who was who. Did my father really look at my own sufferings with the envy and love of someone who already knew himself to be on the other side of an unbridgeable divide? More confusing, even, I'd found out through a review of a biography of Mann in the *Times Literary Supplement* that Mann's bisexuality had been a more or less open secret throughout his life. Despite his traditional and even enduring bourgeois marriage,

his three children, Mann also had several affairs with men. He
had been more daring than his characters.

Seen in this light, from the slightly less pure critical intelligence of the "queer theory" increasingly popular among the
people I was learning to call my colleagues, the last act of Mann's
novella resembles the best-known and most unapologetically "out"
of Mann's stories, *Death in Venice*. Tonio refuses to be drawn
into a bohemian community of other writers and artists and,
rejecting the ambiguous advances of his friend Lizaveta, a Russian painter, travels instead on an unfashionable vacation, a nostalgia journey, to a seaside resort town in what is now Denmark.

He watches the vacationing families at their beach sports
and rich meals; they're unencumbered with any urge to create or
paint or write books, and Tonio admires their raw material health
and wealth, their slightly bovine contentment. One night, at a
hotel dance for the guests that he watches from behind the glazed
doors of the dining room, he sees a man who reminds him of
Hans Hansen, or might be him, in the flesh, grown up, married
to another of the blond Aryan set whom the boy Tonio also had
a crush on.

Watching the couple, he understands that he's at last happy;
his imagination feeds off this feeling of his own estrangement
and longing. He's meant to be the boy alone, outside the gates,
peering through glass windows at the happy couples he never
wants to give up admiring at a distance. *Tonio Kröger* was both
the portrait of an artist as a necessarily alienated and suffering
being, and the portrait of a bisexual, dressed in the costume of a
novelist, alienated most of all from himself.

When I'd finished the *TLS* review, I was almost convinced
that my father hadn't read me *Tonio Kröger* to show me that my
feelings at Riverdale were, as he'd claimed, "normal," or that
what was happening to me at school was something that had already been experienced by Thomas Mann, a century earlier, but
because he'd recognized, in my own eleven-year-old vulnerabil-

ity, an opening in which to plant the seed for a future confession
he'd never have the time or courage to make.

Even as I had this thought, I felt guilty for having it. Thomas
Mann may have slept with young men, but this didn't mean that
my father knew he slept with young men—although it would
have been a strange ignorance. Perhaps, too, my father was drawn
to *Tonio Kröger* not because of its queer subtext but simply for
the fulfillingly unfulfilled life it described. Tonio could not be a
blond, or a horseman, or a Philistine, but he remains forever
faithful to his failure to become one of those people. Perhaps
my father wanted me to remain faithful to the unhappiness I
felt at Riverdale, or perhaps he wanted to say, at the time, that it
was important not to gambol off to some happy country of
liberated sexuality, but to find a strength in ambivalence and
frustration.

"Do not blame this love . . ." Tonio writes to his bohemian
painter friend at the end of the novella, "it is beneficial and fe-
cund; there is longing in it, and a gentle envy, a touch of contempt, and no little innocent bliss." In terms that were not yet
everyday language when Mann wrote that story, Tonio most resembles a voyeur, not a masochist; he has apparently succeeded
in putting himself beyond the touch of physical desire. He didn't
live in a closet but in a room with windows, one of which might,
one day, become a door, although it was impossible to know which
one, or whether he'd stumble, as if by accident, through the window to stand shivering, shard-dusted, bloodied, on the other side.

I'd once brought *Tonio Kröger* with me to the great cathedral-
like reading room of Sterling Library, and I couldn't stop a spasm
of shame that led me to cover the book or place it facedown on
the desk whenever I looked up to glimpse a fellow student or,
worse luck, a professor gliding along the carpeted aisles, arms
laden with what was undoubtedly serious research. I began to

feel that I was in the library under false pretenses, closer kin to the palsied man with a beard and beret who'd flopped himself down once next to me in the reading room and begun to mutter while inscribing exaggerated Kabbalistic notations on a yellow notepad, getting up to grab books off the reference shelves and piling them up until he'd nearly vanished behind them.

I sensed the book I was planning would earn me the immediate contempt of my professors and a fair number of the students. It was not "professional." In an unguarded moment, I'd mentioned something about it to a Russian guy whose comments in our shared seminars I'd always sympathized with. He immediately pronounced the project "deeply disgusting," although he said it half admiringly. A few weeks later, he invited me over for whiskey and read me one of his short stories: bell-like, strange tales often in the voice of a young girl, a complete break from the masterful array of passive moods and dense terminology of his classroom papers.

In comparison with him, I was scarcely capable of subterfuge. I'd already been too explicit about my intention to write about the relations of literature to life, of narrative influence, or, when I remembered to be careful, "the Bourgeois Romantic conceptions of literature and life, with a particular emphasis on scenes of literary consumption and transmission in the works of, for example, Stendhal." My plan to rehabilitate my father had to unfold within this matrix of impersonations, ways of learning to speak that aimed at several audiences at once, as ambiguous and complex as the novels and poems we often analyzed in terms of an author's self-censorship or a society's imposed laws of kosher and unkosher speech acts. We were not supposed to be reading to construct identities but to deconstruct them, to show that what people respond to in literature is not likeness or resemblance, but triggers and codes that lie at an almost molecular level of the brain, immutable laws like those of protein synthesis and DNA transcription. According to such theories, the moments when we think we recognize ourselves are actually the moments when we surrender our agency and are overpowered by the force of those laws, the force of language itself.

Instead of training myself to compete for one of the ever-dwindling number of professorships in the humanities, as if I were running some intellectual marathon, I let my will relax as I read. I grew less interested in discovering some impersonal and scientific-seeming truth of my own about how literature worked, in elaborating and improving upon the estrangement effect of the Russian Formalists, the speech genres and multivoiced negative capability espoused by Bakhtin, or the manipulable laws of form and genre. Nor did I wish to cultivate an aura of expertise, to devote myself to the contents of some dim archive or the life-work of a minor poet or novelist whom I must inevitably claim had been unjustly neglected by the literary establishment of an earlier age. I began to wonder whether the seminar papers we wrote and the monographs we cited revealed actual truths about earlier periods and writers or were merely accounts of those periods and writers reflected through the complex prisms of self-censorship and position jockeying of the contemporary academy where we found ourselves.

In other words, as I complained to my new Russian friend, Kolya, as we emerged from one particularly frustrating class on, as far as we could tell, the ideology of German Romantic landscape gardening, a Goethe novel, and its importance to Walter Benjamin's concept of allegory, I did not exactly want to become a "professor," that is, as I saw it, someone whose job primarily was to act like an enzyme or a host cell in an impersonal process of cultural transmission. It could be thanks to me that people read Shakespeare's late romances or Shelley's poem "Julian and Maddalo," or *Tonio Kröger* in future generations, but ultimately, whether I claimed these texts were among the highest works of art, or documented evolving human friendships over four hundred years, or were merely part of a white male canon of elite

cultural privilege, the important thing was that people continued to hear these names and might grow curious enough to pick
them up for themselves. I had trouble believing I mattered much
to the process, although I supposed I could always have some opposite effect and turn people off from reading, perhaps forever.

We'd ducked into one of the string of local cafés punctuating
the route between the Yale campus and our apartments among the
Victorian and Colonial-style houses of what everyone called the
ghetto. I ordered a brownie, although I said I felt fat. Regardless
of my actual weight, there were more and more days when the
mile and a half walk to and from campus seemed to happen on
a planet with much denser gravity. The sudden rise and fall of
the sugar in my blood, I knew, would shortly act like a cheap and
delicious sedative and knock me out for the rest of the afternoon. We settled on a table, nodding and smiling at nearly everyone, it seemed, hoping, if not for privacy, that we'd be quietly
ignored.

"Do you ever feel like we belong to a generation that will
never do anything?" I asked my new friend.

"You mean we are what Nietzsche would call 'last men,'
people who remain stuck in the old ways without knowing why
they're in the old ways and without being able to change themselves? People whose lives have no meaningful motive apart from
basic human animal wants: food, clothing, shelter, sex."

"Something like that," I agreed. "Everything we do or want
to do comes with an aura of meaninglessness around it. Even
something noble seeming, like going off to do humanitarian
work, or writing a novel, it doesn't matter, they seem shameful,
embarrassing, childlike simulations of things that have already
been done."

I wasn't sure my friend would agree. He'd come to New York
from Moscow when he was sixteen, with barely any English,
and there he was in a PhD program in literature, at one of this
country's best universities. What I'd thought of myself as stum-

bling into, luckily, he must have had to work enormously hard to achieve. Surely his accomplishments made all my meaning-of-life talk seem the complaints of a spoiled child. So I was surprised when he joked that he sometimes missed life under communism; there had been something to fight against, he said, or even something to escape from, or aspire to the promised utopia that never arrived and had gone wrong and needed always to be put right. Without those things to look forward to life was cloudy and dull.

"America," he said, "is like this billboard I saw once when I was visiting Los Angeles. It was an ad for some car and it just said, 'Enjoy Your Drive!' That's what we're all supposed to do. It's like communism but in reverse. There's no state, but all these external private organizations that tell us to be individuals all in the same way."

"Yeah, but what if you don't want to enjoy, or can't?"

"Oh, then there's something wrong with you," he said smilingly, "like Oblomov."

"What?"

"You know the hero, or, rather, antihero of the novel *Oblomov*."

"Of course I know *Oblomov*, my father gave it to me."

"Mine, too," he said.

As we were set to unravel this coincidence, we were distracted by a banging table, the sound of chairs being scraped back against the floor. The noise came from a group of graduate students clustered around two tables pushed together in the corner. One of the student organizers of the movement to unionize graduate teaching assistants was coming down hard on a bunch of first- and second-years who must have been trying to duck out of a meeting or a march:

"Individuals. Everyone here thinks they're an individual," he said. "You know that four out of five of you at this table won't get the tenure-track job you came here for, the job with health care, the job that pays you a living wage, that lets you do the work you came here for, that lets you pay off the loans you might have taken to get here. You know this, you've seen the numbers, but it doesn't matter, because you all think you're number five, the one who's going to make it. That's how they want you to think. The administration will tell you you're the best, you're at Yale, and Yale takes care of you, right, but that's what they say at Harvard, at Duke, at Stanford, and there are a lot of special people out there. I used to be one. They'll make you feel guilty 'cause they're giving you a stipend for two years to do some reading, but then they take that out of your wages, wages they owe you for teaching classes and grading papers for them for the next three or five years. And you'll still feel guilty and think you're special, even when you're driving between your part-time teaching jobs at two community colleges and maybe, if you're lucky, one other college or major university, so you can make ends meet, and hold on until, you tell yourself, you can write that article or book that will get you the job you deserve, that you've been holding out hope for. But where's the time going to come from, when you've got a kid, maybe, or a sick parent, and you're spending the hours that you're not teaching or grading driving or catching up on sleep? And even then, you'll still think you're the one."

One of the listeners excused herself, pushed back her chair, and began walking over to us, taking the chance to escape the call of class consciousness. It was Nastia, also from our class, also, like Kolya, a recent Russian émigrée.

He called after her, exasperated, "You guys are harder to organize than migrant farm workers. It doesn't matter what you got on your SATs, or how smart you are. I could be talking to the next Jacques Derrida or Frederic Jameson or Judith Butler, but if those people were in graduate school now, in the U.S.A., they'd need a union, too, and they'd be smart enough to know it. That's why we've got to support each other, not sit around pretending to be some free-spirited intellectuals from some earlier era."

That last line seemed to float past Nastia as she walked away and landed on me and Kolya, as if to say that he was coming for us next, that this was the last hour of our thoughtless youth. We decided to wave at him. He nodded back and subsided into an apology. This was not how one won friends or influenced people, he knew. The union was going to be our friend, but sometimes friends had to level with you and tell you things you didn't want to know.

As if to confirm our bad influence, Nastia pulled up a chair beside us and sat with her back to the organizer. She asked us to help her decode what the professor, in his lightly accented German English, had meant when he referred to the landscape garden as "a false promise of a perfect reconciliation between man and the natural world," and what he intended by spending nearly the whole last hour of class discussing a single quotation: "He who chooses blindly is struck in the eyes by the smoke of sacrifice." And Kolya and I knew that we'd throw ourselves into it, as if nothing else mattered, as if we were solving a chess problem and in the answer lay a whole understanding of modern tragedy.

Before we began, and more out of politeness, as if wondering whether she'd actually interrupted something more important or interesting than German Romanticism, Nastia asked what we'd been talking about.

"*Oblomov*," I said.

"Oh, *Oblomov*." She sounded relieved. " 'Don't be an Oblomov!' That's what our parents said, right. It's proverbial." At twenty-three, twice married, a favorite of the department chair for her tireless work, her constant attendance at conferences and departmental meetings, Nastia was clearly not an Oblomov.

"I didn't realize American parents gave it to their children, too," she said.

"I think it was just mine," I answered.

But what was an Oblomov, exactly, that one shouldn't be one? I'd begun to wonder. The character's creator, Ivan Goncharov, a civil servant during the reformist decades of Alexander II, had certainly believed he was writing a scientific novel, a diagnostic study anatomizing the laziness and terminal ennui afflicting the Russian nobility of the middle nineteenth century. When I'd first tried to read the novel, after my father had offered it to me sometime in my senior year of high school, I couldn't even get beyond the first forty pages: our man, an aristocratic landowner living on his rents, was still in bed, still in his bathrobe, still calling for his manservant, Zakhar, to get him dressed. After forty pages! Life was too short.

In the emptier New Haven days, when I was more concerned with slowing time down, I pushed through my boredom to discover that he stays in bed for another ten pages, followed by thirty more of Oblomov trying to get dressed and another thirty over the course of which he tries to leave his rented apartment in Moscow, and is instead besieged by a host of fake friends who've been ripping him off. Seeing no way out, he falls back asleep and dreams of his overprotected childhood on his ancestral village estate. The author was proving his point, maybe too well. At last, arriving on the scene to get Oblomov out of the house and get the novel moving, comes Oblomov's childhood friend, Stoltz. The half-German son of the Oblomov family's estate manager, Stoltz starts out as an equal and opposite caricature: the modern nineteenth-century man of action, he's an encyclopedic collector of the latest facts, a devotee of gymnastics, and an enthusiast for the latest revolutionary farming technologies. Farming technology is pretty much the only revolutionary thing about him. He doesn't want to shoot his childhood friend and former playmate; instead he proposes a diet and offers to take him on the travels he's planning to collect even more facts and experiences.

The two friends then engage in one of those long debates that seem to be written down only in Russian novels and Platonic dialogues, although they still occur among just about everyone who understands themselves to be free and capable of a conscious decision about how to live a good life. The debate in

Oblomov is somewhat one-sided, since it's hard to credit the cakes, ale, and sunburned, plump, bare-armed peasant girls Oblomov summons to defend his view that, since the purpose of life is to gain enough money to be able to relax in sensual peace, and he's already got that, then his life was already over before it began. All he can do is more of the same; so why do anything, he wonders. Stoltz calls this attitude "Oblomovitis." And it's easy enough for him to prove to his old friend that Oblomov himself doesn't really believe what he's arguing, that underneath the sensualist lies a man with ambitions and hopes similar in nature, though not in exact form, to Stoltz's own, ambitions and hopes that only need an opportunity to escape the stifling weight of aristocratic laziness.

This, it seemed, is about as far as most Russian parents expect their children to get in the novel, although we're nearly two hundred pages in by that point. Oblomov is successfully shamed out of his laziness, at least for the length of the scene. He knows he's being ridiculous, but neither Oblomov nor Stoltz, nor Goncharov, their author, really knows why he acts that way. Oblomovitis is not a coherent worldview, and Oblomov doesn't even pretend it is. The disease is about more than "class" or fat, decadent aristocrats. Tolstoy was also an aristocrat, and no one would accuse him of idleness or ennui. If anything, Oblomovitis seems like a psychological condition, but of what kind?

As I read on to the end, I discovered a quite different novel inside the didactic one, a novel that totally escapes the sound moral and medical intentions of its author and of readers who think their children just need a stern warning against laziness and pernicious ideologies.

For one thing, the novel turns into one of the weirder love triangles in literary history: Stoltz takes Oblomov to meet the girl he secretly intends to marry as soon as he's made a name for himself: bright, musical, shy Olga Ilyinsky, daughter of a recently impoverished aristocratic family. Almost as a test for her, not of her fidelity but of her capacity for kindness and selflessness, he charges her with looking after Oblomov, cheering him up, getting him to take an interest in life again. She begins to do this by playing and singing Oblomov's favorite opera aria for him. Not just a common pastime for any class with access to instruments, music was also one of the treatments the nineteenth century prescribed for melancholics. Oblomov responds with an awestruck silence she mistakes for criticism. As he fumbles around, trying to fix this embarrassing misimpression, Oblomov turns brave, for once, and ends up telling Olga what she soon realizes are the first sincere compliments paid her by any man. No other man she knows is capable of speaking about his feelings and impressions as well as Oblomov, in part because he thinks of himself as an invalid more than as a man.

Stoltz takes Oblomov's sudden pride in his appearance and his renewed interest in music and poetry as evidence that his planned treatment is working, and he leaves Oblomov and Olga together while he goes off on a European business trip, writing to Oblomov to meet him in Paris in a few weeks. "It's now or never," he tells him. Unsurprisingly, Oblomov doesn't go anywhere, although the novel stays mute on whether his inertia is only a relapse of the old Oblomovitis, as Stoltz tells him it is, or a sign that he's actually fallen in love with Olga and she with him. When Stoltz returns several months later, Olga and Oblomov are engaged.

Out of this mess of a didactic novel, a curiously complicated portrait of desires was starting to emerge. Even setting aside my own doubly triangulated and heavily, shamefully interested reading of the novel, a reading in which I was simultaneously wondering if I was going to turn out to be an Oblomov, or if my father had turned out to be one, I also wondered whether Oblomov himself was going to escape the fate his cruel author had prepared for him. His courtship scenes with Olga possess a gentle awkwardness and unforced tenderness, as if the author were merely standing by, allowing things to unfold while forgetting that the novel might have somewhere to go, a plot, a motive. "This novel too suffers from Oblomovitis," I wrote in the margin. Actions get distended over weeks and months. Stealing one's best friend's almost-fiancée should seem fraught, but it comes out muddled, an accident more than a moral outrage.

Oblomov does not escape his fate. The author cannot be that capricious. But Goncharov is also keen to establish that Oblomov and Olga have some sort of real and untainted affection for each other. He succeeds so well that it's unclear whether their love is ultimately doomed because neither of them is yet a finished, whole person with an independent sense of his or her qualities and worth, or whether Oblomov, for all the flaws rendering him unfit for the bustling, modern middle classes, finally achieves a limited heroic self-consciousness. It's possible that he understands how he's undermined his only friend's happiness and so decides to sacrifice himself for Stoltz's sake as well as Olga's. Or it might be that he feels both are too good for him. This worshipful attitude comes out most clearly in Nikita Mikhalkov's Soviet-era film adaptation. Under cover of an official Marxist historical drama about pre-Soviet decadence, Mikhalkov's movie comes across as more sympathetic to Oblomov than Goncharov might have liked. His camera adopts Oblomov's point of view, always reclining or seated, always looking up at Stoltz or Olga from below, often catching them backlit in some aura of natural light, making them seem larger and brighter, burnished in the view of an adoring child.

It's also unclear whether Oblomov's surrender is at all something he intends. He's already too habituated to oversleeping his own life. His love for Olga doesn't permanently change any of the habits he had before, but neither does his accidental and unknowing betrayal of Stoltz make him hard or cruel. Oblomov simply withdraws from what might have been his life. He puts off the marriage until he can get his estate in order, which he never quite manages to do; he rents rooms in a dilapidated house in a quiet Moscow suburb where he's ashamed to let Olga visit him. Again and again, by intention or irrational action, he disappoints her until she's led inevitably back to Stoltz. Meanwhile he begins an affair with his landlady, a relative of one of his disreputable sponging false friends, but a good soul who answers to the fantasy of the pie-baking, sunburned peasants of his childhood.

This was hardly the stuff of high tragedy, but it was incredibly sad; I could feel its sadness surfacing in me precisely because the novel always stops short of melodramatic action, just as the lives I knew had always stopped just before tipping over into something really awful—unless the really awful thing was stopping just short of the awful but close enough to see it.

I broke down completely at the epilogue, when Stoltz, now married to Olga, returns to look for his friend and finds that he, too, has got married, although only in secret, to the landlady of the plump arms, as the book calls her, and they're raising their son in the little suburban house, a picture of quiet contentment and stasis: "at midday a clerk's elegant high heels clattered along the pavement, a muslin curtain in some window moved aside, and the wife of some civil servant peeped out from behind the geraniums." Oblomov, "the complete natural reflection and expression of that repose that reigned all around him," is, at last, a real invalid, having had the first of the heart attacks that will eventually end him. "I know everything and understand everything," he tells Stoltz, before sending him on his way forever. "I have, for a long time, been ashamed to live in the world."

Stoltz persists on calling this attitude Oblomovitis, even to the very end, as if it helped. But Oblomov's own words seem a more accurate diagnosis of his condition: he suffers from a persistent and unshakable feeling of shame, a shame whose origin the novel never reveals. Laziness and irresolution, the ease with which he gives up his ambitions for his own life, all these are only opportunistic symptoms of Oblomov's real disease, not the disease itself. While Goncharov and the Russian reformers and parents who came after him were right to urge their children not to be Oblomovs, it was far from certain that Oblomov—or anyone else who'd fallen under the spell of this primal shame—could really do much about it.

Was this, instead of any didactic message, what my father had been trying to tell me? Had my father suffered from Oblomovitis before contracting any actual disease? In what was starting to seem a slightly mad method, I let myself superimpose the novel on my father's life and my own to see what changed, what news it could bring me. If my father was an Oblomov, if, more important, he saw himself as an Oblomov, that is to say someone suffering from a deep and ineradicable sense of shame, what could this tell me about how he'd organized his life, our common life, before it fell apart? Did that make my mother Olga, the musician, or Agafya, the pie-baking landlady from a lower class whose lower-classness ultimately remains her most prominent feature, regardless of her virtues? The question sounded stupid to me, even as I couldn't help wondering about it. People are not characters in some sort of one-to-one correspondence. Yet it was only by asking questions like these that I had any hope of finding out how it might have felt to have been my father, and how he might have understood his relationships to other people and to the world.

Through the novel I was able to remember a forgotten story of my parents' early courtship, one of the few they had both told me. It involved one of the rare occasions when my father had taken my mother to meet his father, in an Upper East Side restaurant. My mother described how she'd found what she thought was the perfect dress, black with white ruffles at the sleeves and neck. As they got into a taxi heading uptown from the West Village, where they lived then, he told her she looked like a waitress from Schrafft's, a chain of ice cream parlor cafés that now exists only as a low-end supermarket brand of oversized ice cream tubs. In my father's childhood, however, it was a posher Starbucks of its day, just as Starbucks will probably be the Schrafft's of some future. My mother was, as she said, completely humiliated by the comparison; she'd refused to go into the restaurant until they'd stopped and bought a sweater she could put over what she could then only think of as a waitress's uniform.

As I imagined the scene in the Oblomovian light of my reading, it came to seem something entirely typical of my family of Oblomovs. My father had protested that he hadn't meant to be condescending or insulting, he was only saying what came to his mind when he saw my mother in the dress. This was just how it was, as he saw it. Who knows, perhaps he'd even fantasized about the Schrafft's waitresses the way Oblomov fantasized about the house serfs in his family's kitchen. To my mother, my father's remark showed her she was dressing in a way his family would see as the dress of a servant. He knew his father would look down on my mother and on him, that there was something shaming about the whole episode, and what my father thought of as a neutral-sounding observation, my mother probably rightly heard as an accusation: she was going to embarrass my father because she was making him feel like his fiancée was a Schrafft's waitress.

I realized my father had always lived in terror of embarrassment. This old-country shame culture could rise up at any moment. The accusations he'd leveled while disinheriting me mostly had to do with moments when I'd done something embarrassing, either to him or myself: making a fuss about my black babysitter in a way that made her think my parents were racists, getting pee on the floor while we were guests of a psychoanalyst friend, who would see this as evidence of some poignant parental failure, or my playing conspicuous air piano during a house concert in a way that might lead the pianist to think our family made fun of her behind her back and that I was merely imitating my parents' imitations. It occurred to me, then, that part of the reason he often refused to attend my concerts and plays was that he was more afraid of the embarrassment he might feel if I were to mess up than enticed by the happier thought that I might do well. For all his high talk, or alongside his high talk about culture and the duty to oppose Philistinism, he felt that life itself was nothing but a series of opportunities to behave shamefully, a series of potential humiliations, and this feeling, along with *Oblomov*, the novel that tried to embarrass a society out of its embarrassment, had been passed down to me.

If my aunt had been right, which my mother had told me she wasn't, then my father really did have a referent or reason to feel that he was always on the point of being discovered in some shameful act, even when he and everyone associated with him behaved with perfect grace. Like *Tonio Kröger*, the script of *Oblomov* could be reworked as an account of someone who understood, even unconsciously, that to give in to his greatest desires would mean an end to his participation in the only society he'd ever known. Everything he'd been used to having over the years would no longer be available to him, all the more because that world worked by always offering a petty enjoyment, a substitute satisfaction, in exchange for surrendering your highest and most dangerous desires. What was worse, it seemed all too easy to spend one's life hard at work, like Stoltz and not like Oblomov, but only to create a false life that simultaneously kept out the true life you fantasized about, driving that life underground and allowing it to exist untouched and underdeveloped, in secret.

If my aunt was right, then our domestic life and my father's professional life, no matter how seriously he took them, were only like the sets of Venetian blinds we used over our windows at the Central Park West apartment. No matter how much you tried shutting them, thin rays of light shone through. The world outside was never hidden completely, but made up of these overlapping bands of light and dark.

But I was convinced my aunt had gone too far in her suspicions. In the account she gave of their childhood, my father was never good enough because he'd been born into a circle of hell, the unloved offspring of an unloving marriage. And that feeling itself, of general inadequacy, more than anything he thought about or did, could have been enough to infect several lives. In the evidence I had from my own life, there was so much to be ashamed of, always, that the feeling of general guilt and shame could have easily got peeled away from any actual forbidden longing. Guilt was our habit. It might as well have been original sin. A sense of being always in the wrong followed us around.

11

Having scribbled versions of my thoughts on *Tonio Kröger* and *Oblomov* into a soft brown-covered notebook, which I'd labeled "My Father's Library," my thinking came to a halt. I suppose I might have even been dimly aware of what at times—in terms my colleagues would have understood—felt like "hermeneutic anxiety." In more ordinary English, I worried that if I approached these books as if they contained, in buried code, the answer to the question of what my father had really desired from his maimed life, I would only find the very answer I was looking for evidence against.

In other words, my selection, even though they were books that my father had selected himself, was already too partial to my aunt's version of events to provide a strong enough counter-narrative, the kind that my mother might have liked to read: about his dedication to finding a vaccine for malaria, about the rise of a scientific and evenhanded temperament in a man who'd devoted himself to fashioning the best possible life imaginable, not just for himself and his family, but also for humanity as a whole. Had his illness stripped the dignity not only from his body but from his life as well, and could anyone ever give that back?

Another fear was that I was merely being self-indulgent, socially irresponsible, and politically incorrect. I was twenty-six years old, had added nothing to the world. The union organizers had caught up to me eventually, sat me down, and persuaded me to become involved in the struggle for greater equality, at least among academics. I'd been "organized," as they said. My arguments about all greater change beginning locally were ready to be tested on incoming graduate students from backgrounds as wealthy as my own. They made sense to me, but I had no illusions that I was doing it for myself. I did it, really, despite myself, and that attitude of doing things despite myself seemed to me the best reason to engage in politics, not to get what I wanted but to make it easier for others to get what they needed. It was the right thing to do because a part of me seemed always to rebel against doing the right thing.

And then, one night, though not much less drunk, only less impaired, than a few of the British contingent, I'd been chauffeuring them back to their respective houses. Last on the drop-off list, it happened, was a girl who, earlier that evening, had taken me aside on the balcony where a bunch of us were smoking and told me she was glad I wasn't the arrogant tosser I'd seemed like during our one shared seminar. When I'd double-parked the car in front of her house, she invited me up for a nightcap, "at which point," she added, "you'll really be too drunk to drive." I accepted. The next morning she somewhat guiltily went with me to the tow pound to retrieve my car. I drove her home and she invited me up again. She reminded me to park properly.

It was the start of something, but a something that seemed impossible to reconcile with my relationship to my father's books. What could this person have seen in me that made me worth desiring? And how had she known that I'd always found her fascinating, albeit in a slightly forbidding way, that I'd stolen the wine at the department party in part to impress her? What would she do when she discovered that I was pursuing my embarrassing and irresponsible reading? I would have to hide it from her, or maybe better give it up completely. My growing closeness to my father threatened to make any present love impossible. And yet,

like a teenager who couldn't stop looking in the mirror, I yearned
for and dreaded every moment I spent among my father's books.
They yielded so many moments of recognition that I couldn't
help feeling they must mean something, point somewhere.

There was an afternoon when I found my own disinheritance again in the pages of *The Way of All Flesh*, the lightly fictionalized memoirs of Samuel Butler, a multifaceted fuck-up of
a man, maybe best known for arguing, in 1897, that the *Odyssey*
had been written by a woman. The first proud atheist from a
family of clergymen that stretched back generations, he was also
a critic of Darwin's theory of evolution, and was fascinated by
the inheritance of behavior rather than genes. About the same
time that a certain Viennese doctor was publishing his first case
studies of hysteria, Butler began his autobiographical novel with
his great-grandfather's family, setting out a portrait of three generations of family unhappiness, a period lasting from the end of
the eighteenth century to the dawn of the twentieth.

It was a book my father wanted me to read at sixteen, but, in
a different way from *Oblomov*'s slowness, I'd found too bleak
and glacially paced. What patience my father had with these interminable nineteenth-century and pre-Modernist, early-twentieth-
century novels! What patience the writers of these novels must
have had, what quantities of time and energy! The length and
ponderous steps of the sentences, their heightened and euphemis-
tic tone had penetrated through to me, almost becoming the only
idiom of my thoughts as I read them. Really this language belonged to some age before the creation of the reserve army of intellectual labor of which I was a part. They spoke of a time free
of the constant barrage of competing demands on our attention, a time when the signals transmitted across generations burst
through with greater clarity and insistence, before they were
drowned out by the incessant *pip-pip-pip*s of present stimulation.

A century and ten years too late, I came across a scene in
which Butler finds a letter from his grandfather to his father,

written at a moment when his father hesitates to become an An-
glican priest: "You mistake your own mind, and are suffering
from a nervous timidity which may be very natural but may not
the less be pregnant with serious consequences to yourself. I am
not at all well, and the anxiety occasioned by your letter is naturally preying on me. You shall not receive a single sixpence from
me until you come to your senses," the grandfather writes. Later,
of course, this cowed son will take the chance to disinherit his
own child once he, too, tests the limits of his independence of
mind and action.

If only I had read this at sixteen! What might I have been
spared? Would I have been forearmed enough to say at the moment of crisis, "Dad, stop playing *The Way of All Flesh* with me.
We've both read the book. We know how it turns out; how it
leads to blocked, shriveled lives, how the unjust exercise of power
leads to more unjust exercises of power, age after age. Don't do
it." If I could have spoken to my father as he spoke to me, in this
language of books already written, would he have stopped, reined
himself in even though he was not at all well, spoken to me honestly, man to man instead of father to son?

How much power I'd had, and hadn't even known it. But
that very power assumed my father had had some dim inkling of
what he was ultimately capable of three years before he did it.
How often had he fantasized about threatening me? His reasons
for handing me that book and all the other ones were probably
as vague and impalpable to him as they'd been to me. I supposed that's why I'd sidestepped them, out of a self-preserving
ignorance.

Stepping back into this canon of disappointment and unhappiness, I'd somehow begun again to take on my father; not
just wrestling with him or confronting him, but also submitting
myself to a process of willing transformation that weakened
whatever there was of me that stood apart from him. If I was
having such trouble distilling my father's sense of himself from

these narratives, it was perhaps because my sense of myself had become hopelessly knotted up with my father's, and the behavior and habits revealed in the pages. Everything there spoke to me of an unavoidable doom of thwarted desire, tarnished hope, a practice of disappointment to which I felt already too thoroughly habituated.

I hated him, again, or maybe I really hated him for the first time. It didn't matter what my father had done or not done in the hours when he wasn't being my father. What mattered was what he'd done to me: his obscure injunctions to read this or that, to be my own person as long as I was never disappointing or embarrassing him or watching televised sports, or playing the wrong music, or reading the wrong books, or failing to use a condom, or going to the wrong college, or saying Kaddish at his funeral. Why did I still feel such loyalty to the old tyrant, and to my mother for enabling his peculiar regime? My education in unhappiness seemed almost designed to stub my existence into a cycle of joyless, half-finished, poisoned encounters.

The father I'd restored to life through my clandestine reading was less mystifying and terrifying than the one I'd known as a child, but this only made things worse. He was somehow smaller, more mediocre, pitiable at best, in the way that Theobald Pontifex, the awful father of *The Way of All Flesh*, is shown to be only a mediocre clergyman saddled with a ridiculous name. Perhaps this was an improvement in things, at least from a certain psychological standpoint. Better not to say, with all the melodrama appropriate to an earlier age, "Family, I hate you!" but only with the faded dismissiveness of my own, "Family, you suck!"

And yet I wasn't wholly persuaded by the idea that families sucked in general, although it might be better to think about all the rest of life that happened outside anything like family. Nor really was I ready to accept that my family sucked in its own particular way. Things had gone wrong for us. That was true. But did it have to be like that? "You might try imagining your parents loved you," my girlfriend said to me, a few months later. We were packing up to visit her mother in England, a prelude to our summer plan of renting a small house in Oxford. And whatever nervousness I had about living with this person vanished with her words, echoing C's earlier ones to me. They confirmed that we were right for each other. She was going to write her dissertation on a genre she called "tragic overliving," while I converted my notes into something like a book, a memoir of reading, the promised countermemoir against my aunt. I told her I'd try.

I'd slipped Turgenev's *Fathers and Sons* into my carry-on bag, in the unavoidable Penguin Classics edition. It was the last of the novels on my list, and I was determined to carry through my reading without much hope that I'd receive any definitive answer in it. Unlike the other novels, I thought I knew *Fathers and Sons* quite well, and I'd chosen it not because of the title, which sounds overloaded to contemporary ears, but because of the death of Bazarov, the modern man of science, nihilist, and country doctor, around whom the other characters flutter like moths to light.

He goes to perform an autopsy on a peasant who has died of typhus, cuts himself, and becomes infected in turn. The wound is cauterized too late and the remedy, in the days before antibiotics, was bound to be ineffectual in any case. It was one of the rare instances I could recall of a death in literature that so closely matched the manner of what I believed to be my father's own, even as Bazarov's first name, Evgeny, was the Russian version of my father's. I tried not to think about the coincidence, but, once I noticed it, I could only put it at the back of my mind, at best. Presumably my father, too, had had this stirring of recognition, had succumbed to the weak illusion of identification. I remembered the scenes of Bazarov's ending quite well, but I was no longer sure when exactly I'd read the novel, or how my father had got it into my hands.

Random death, whether in fiction or in life, appears to violate a basic sense that a person's actions and principles should
have some sort of meaning in relation to the story as a whole.
Bazarov's ordinary, random stupidity, although perfectly realis-
tic, breaks whatever illusion of realism most people come to expect from a character-driven novel of family or social life. Almost
like saying "and then he woke up." The reader is left with a heap
of tangled loose ends: Bazarov has just wounded his friend's
uncle after the older man challenges him to a duel; he may or
may not compromise his nihilist principles and marry; he could
become a full-fledged modern revolutionary, or just a country
doctor, like his own father. All these outcomes remain forever
suspended in the reader's mind.

This brazenly antinovelistic gesture felt truer or braver to me
than the explanation-haunted backgrounds of the other novels
I'd chosen to speak for my father: the predestined alienation of
the artistic temperament in *Tonio Kröger*, the acquired shame of
Oblomov, or the inherited violence of *The Way of All Flesh*.
Whether he knew it or not, Turgenev seems to be exposing the
limitations of certain literary modes of understanding character
and fate, or, in a sly way, suggesting that these literary modes are
anachronisms of an earlier age when novelistic sensibility could
still make sense of the world. There's a scene in which Bazarov's
younger friend and protegé, Arkady Kirsanov, takes a volume of
Pushkin out of his father's hands and replaces it with a German
textbook on modern agriculture, *Material and Power*. Arkady's
uncle, Pavel Petrovich, the aristocratic aesthete who takes it upon
himself to defend the traditional sentiments behind the Russian
aristocratic order against Bazarov's arguments, reads English
novels, speaks French, quotes poetry, and has chosen to live his
life in a kind of stylized mourning for a youthful and unconsum-
mated love affair, a widowed bachelor. The mixture of sentimentalism and selfishness in this type of literary sensibility were flaws
Turgenev also seemed to have noted in himself.

Yet, even if Bazarov's death proves his view of the world to be more accurate than that of the sentimental novelist who created him, Turgenev at least succeeds in aestheticizing nihilism. The blow Bazarov refers to as his "unfortunate incident" is also thoroughly, suspiciously, in character—as scientific, arbitrary, and nihilistic as the doctrines he espouses. If he doesn't get what he deserves, exactly, he at least gets a death he can rationalize—a victim of the unsanitary conditions and ignorance of the Russian countryside that he would change if he could.

Among nihilists, in literature or in life, Bazarov is not a ferocious or even dangerous specimen. His nihilism doesn't require terrorism or random acts of violence. It is not a philosophy of action, only a refusal to believe in anything beyond the evidence of the senses. He dissects frogs but is otherwise kind to animals; treats rich and poor alike. He seems to have no fixed principles except an embrace of absurdity; he even binds the wound of Pavel Petrovich after he reluctantly shoots him in their duel. He urges Arkady to reconcile with his father at the beginning of the novel, both in the interests of science, to see how the old guard is adapting to recent land reforms, but also, as he says, so the young man won't become one of those bad-faith liberals, living off the rents of an estate he avoids so as not to embarrass his revolutionary convictions. His own parents he treats well—he's their only child—while they worry about driving him away through an excess of affection.

When it comes to families, *Fathers and Sons* turns out to be, in fact, one of the rare nineteenth-century novels of essentially happy ones. There are no plausible motives for parricide, as in *The Brothers Karamazov*, no violent inheritance quarrels, no love affairs or bitter rivalries for limited affections and resources across generations or between siblings and friends, although Turgenev makes sure to float a ghost of each of these possible outcomes at points when the novel seems to be slowing into a pastoral fantasy. Arkady's father has just had another son with his former house serf when the novel opens, but, despite Bazarov's provoking insinuations, Arkady feels no deep rivalry or fear, and even wants his father to make his second marriage legitimate. Such resistance to melodrama allows another kind of action to become central to the novel: how members of families learn to see each other as independent beings with separate lives, not with the resigned sense of giving up influence—"Oh, he's his own person"—but really as a form of active understanding and thinking about the independent lives of those closest to us.

To get at this sense of intergenerational reconciliation, Turgenev structures the novel adroitly around the rather banal-seeming act of inviting a friend for an extended visit with one's family. First Bazarov is the guest of the Kirsanovs on their estate and then Arkady stays with Bazarov in the village where his father is the resident doctor. This simple device forces the family to appear within society, or at least under some benevolently objectifying perspective, rather than as a private refuge where one's least social impulses hold sway. The presence of an interested questioner also permits certain feelings to come out that would otherwise be suppressed. Hearing a Schubert cello melody fill the Kirsanov house, Bazarov can ask the reader's question, "Who's playing?" and when Arkady replies that it's his father, Bazarov then starts to laugh at him, "a paterfamilias of forty-four, in this out of the way district, playing on the violincello." At that moment, Arkady, for all his own burgeoning nihilist tendencies and student distrust of sentimentalism, realizes that he actually likes that his father plays the cello and has no wish to ban cello playing or Schubert from his nihilist republic.

Likewise, under Arkady's guileless questioning while the two friends smoke in the hayloft, Bazarov admits that he, too, loves his parents and that he's undeniably the center of all their hopes for the future. The novel seems to exist for the sake of making such banal scenes feel almost miraculous. Through scenes like these, Turgenev appears to assert a subtle case for his liberal aesthetic view of life. If only people understood each other as full characters, then all this talk of nihilism versus patriarchy, of one generation against another, or one man against another would simply become fading background noise at a dinner party. There are no conflicts, only pseudo-conflicts and misperceptions, as when Bazarov mistakenly thinks Arkady is wooing a woman he isn't even sure he loves himself. Instead, Arkady is pursuing her younger sister, in perfect keeping with a law of symmetry in which like is attracted to like and there's enough for everyone. Only inevitable death shadows the blissful kermess of generations, and even Bazarov's death, cruel and capricious as it is, appears like a strangely willed naïveté on the part of the novelist. Had Bazarov not cut himself while dissecting the corpse, he could have only either advanced his nihilism to the bomb-throwing stage the movement reached a few years later with the assassination of Alexander II, or inherited his father's place as a well-meaning but essentially powerless country doctor in a semifeudal order.

Unlike the other novels in my canon, I had trouble recognizing my family among either the Bazarovs or the Kirsanovs. There was a quality to the relationships in *Fathers and Sons* that I could only think of as "postadolescent," the very stage my family and I had not reached intact. Even when I was a teenager there had been few third parties, outsiders to my parents' world who I could speak to, who knew me and them and could bring me to an admission that I still loved my mother's piano playing and missed it. The only one, really, was C, and *Fathers and Sons* seemed more like the kind of book that suited her vision of the world. As my girlfriend had suggested, I could imagine that my parents loved me, but their love felt different from the parental love in the book, more aggressive and impatient. It seemed they were waiting for me to return from a journey into adulthood that I hadn't yet undertaken, expecting me to be prefortified with Arkady's strong liberal emotions of tolerance, pity mixed with tenderness mixed with embarrassment mixed with belief in the fundamental all-rightness of family life.

Had my father given me the novel in order to try to hasten me there, to push me into a kind of emotional precociousness as he'd once pushed me to memorize French poetry, to try to outwit the dread Oedipal complex he believed in despite himself? I tried to remember how he'd given the book to me. Was it one morning, on or about my sixteenth birthday, my father, in a rare moment of halting advance, knocking at the door of my bedroom, still in the paisley-silk bathrobe, his dressing gown—he was such an Oblomov!—limping cautiously across the chesslike parquet squares, taking in the teenage funk, the hockey stick in the corner, the Afghan girl photo on the corkboard, the magazines and science fiction books piled on the windowsill, thinking, "How on earth will this experiment work?", extending the gift in the darkish green wrapping paper that we offered to shoppers at Shakespeare & Co.—was that it?

That didn't seem right at all. My mother usually gave me presents, and the green wrapping paper was from the summer, one year later, when I'd worked at the bookstore, although my aunt too had sometimes given me books from Shakespeare & Co., before she switched allegiance to the new Barnes and Noble, which also, I remembered, used green wrapping paper. Perhaps the whole wrapping-paper image was a false lead. My blankness, my inability to turn up the precise moment of transmission, upset me. Nor could I remember whether my father and I had even discussed the book; although I was pretty sure I'd read it while he was still alive, I was beginning to doubt even that. So many other memories had returned to me undiminished, as I read those other novels, to the point that I really did feel I'd regained my father, or at least a version of him, though not one I was at all happy with. Yet, somehow, at the moment when I'd found the novel that came closest to confirming my father's own words and my mother's belief in an absolute familial fount of benevolence, I remembered nothing.

I didn't read *Fathers and Sons* on the plane to England, but saved it up for what felt like a suitable space of reflection. That space turned out to be the main reading room of the Bodleian Library at Oxford, the original that the Yale library palely copied. I'd obtained entrance on my graduate-student credentials— pretending to do some research on a dissertation topic involving British Romanticism that I'd dreamed up before I left New Haven—and a letter vouching for my scholarly intentions from my girlfriend's mother, an Oxford professor. I swore the traditional oath about obeying all library rules before the kindly seeming Scottish woman of light burr and large-framed glasses, and though I wasn't going to steal books or light fires or plagiarize, the swearing ceremony brought back that same sense of my being a fraud that I'd felt in the Yale library. There I was, tunneling underneath the edifice of scholarship after some genuine, personal connection, and I couldn't even remember how I'd first come into possession of the novel I was relying on to provide me with a sense of the truth.

If my father had read *Fathers and Sons* at all, he'd read it as I was reading it at that moment, as fiction, a plausible-seeming arrangement of events, even if that arrangement turned out to be false or to falsify something about certain families just as they accurately reflected others. I began to understand, as perhaps I ought to have right away, that I was probably not going to find a definitive answer to the insinuations my aunt had whispered throughout the pages of her memoir. Certainly I wasn't going to discover anything absolute about my father beyond certain feelings for his literary tastes. While I was never going to be able to win through and determine what desires exactly motivated those tastes, my reading had at least brought me to a point where my father's life seemed more richly ambiguous to me than what was implied by "Husband, Father, Scientist." Nor could I say that he "loved" these books, or what it meant to be a man who loved books. He, and now I, had both come to need these books. They'd taken the place of friends, companions, and families. They'd become the guests we'd invited to visit us, in the solitude of our family estates. But what they made us see was not some bright truth, only something like the molecular form of a desire whose trace we carried within us, the parasite in the garden. No cure seemed possible.

I got up from my place, gathered up my brown-covered notebook, pencil, and novel, and wandered out, dazed, into the courtyard, and began to walk into the rare sun of an English June, past the gated garden closes of colleges, past roaring busloads of American kids on summer programs, down along a canal bank, past cows, past drunks, past quiet lives on houseboats, past my past, remote, unwinnable.

Eventually I stopped at a pub, for lunch, a beer. The European soccer championships were on. I watched the French team in elegant blues as they, too, passed, though with purpose, running with forceful assurance, an ease of discipline, "Deschamps, Lizarazu, Deschamps, Thuram, Petit, Deschamps, Wiltord," the announcer called, voice rising in excitement with each pass, as if the ability to weave an unbroken series of names was itself a triumph. I lost myself in the game for a while, as I used to as a child when frustrated, the perfectly completed nothingness of beautiful boredom, satisfaction in the hard work of others. There was a touch of contempt, a gentle longing, and no little innocent bliss.

I got up and walked myself back to the covered market, bought strawberries, a fresh cheese, some greens, vaguely intending dinner. My memory did not return. My girlfriend announced she'd written ten pages. I hid my jealousy with offers of a movie. The local art house cinema was showing something summery and French. We got on our bicycles and rode, she with the lightness of someone going to a just reward, while I swerved, distracted, making sure to remember to stay on the correct, English side of the road. Later, sleepless, smoking in the little garden of our rented cottage, listening to the peculiar sound of snails scrunching leaves in the underbrush, amid the night quiet, I felt like a strangely fortunate person, to be so loved by another on grounds obscure to myself. I owed it to her not to be stuck in the past but to move forward with her, even if she was now ahead of me by yards, the way she'd been that evening when we pedaled to the theater. I'd been acting as if ordinary time did not apply to me, as if I could remain enthralled, scrutinizing my father's books as I'd stood reading his gravestone while the world wheeled on without me. Each day moved me ever farther from the possibility of recovering the lost and forgotten hours of my childhood, of filling in the gaps of what might never have been there at all. If my private reading had done some things to bring me a sense of my father's "textuality," as I jokingly thought of it, it seemed to have done little to help me understand my own.

In my blind search and furious frozen contemplation there had been such a wealth of things around me I'd missed. It occurred to me that I didn't have to feel like such a complete phony in the library if I actually honored the place and used it the way it was more or less intended: as a space of devotion to other voices from other pasts, not my own. Why not transport myself to some other tradition, one not native to me, where my mind could take root and grow again in open curiosity, bad seed made good? Why not view the marble blankness of my family life as some kind of happy accident that pushed me out into a much wider world than I would otherwise have reached?

In the weeks that followed, I returned to the library and filled out call slips for the books listed on what I still thought of as my fake proposal. When my girlfriend asked how the book about my father was going, I'd say it was moving along, which seemed to satisfy her, or I'd change the subject to her work, or my excitement at having discovered that Stendhal actually had met the English critic William Hazlitt in Paris, in 1824. Sometimes, I'd wake up in the night, restless with the sense of something left undone, a voice that told me I'd left the lights on, the door unlocked, the gas stove lit. Then I'd sit down with the brown notebook and go over what I'd written, as if I'd missed something in my sentences that would allow me to recover the swirling momentum of emotions that had pitched me into this maze: reading my father reading.

Weeks lengthened into years. When we returned from Oxford, the notebook went into an old steamer trunk I used to store letters, files, photographs, the fragments of all my incoherent past episodes. I was thinking that one day, perhaps, if I had more time, these would suddenly reveal themselves in some fuller light of more perfect understanding. Until that day, I'd go on, as I had before, carrying this sense of something incomplete within me.

12

Recently, on the nights when my five-year-old daughter sleeps at my apartment, she's taken to asking me about my childhood. "Tell me a story about when you were in kindergarten," she demands, usually right before she's supposed to be going to bed and we're lying in the dark in the room that doubles as my office and her bedroom. When she was three and I'd first moved into the apartment—during what I told myself was a temporary separation while her mother and I were working things out at the marriage counselor's—I'd called it a dingy building, on account of the moldy smell, peeling paint, the worn brown rug on the windowless staircase leading up from the entryway. My daughter picked up the word and, when missing her mother, or out of nothing other than shared aesthetic feeling, would say to me, "I don't want to go to your apartment; it's dingy."

I quite liked my dingy apartment, at least the nondingy parts. It had been carved out of what was formerly some family's sunroom, an enclosed terrace on the top floor, six ancient and chipped casement windows wide and three casement windows long, reached after a quick walk down the long narrow entrance corridor, ignoring the smaller bedroom on the left, separated from the main space by flimsy drywall. The whole occupied a rear-wing extension of a row house on a block of seemingly identical row houses. Thanks to this extension, a glorious violation of the pitiless planning of most Philadelphia blocks, my apartment jutted out at least fifteen feet beyond the surrounding buildings into their quiet back gardens.

I came to cherish the extra space, almost an extra dimension, which lent the place a green and private feel. Sunlight poured in at all daylight hours over the rooftops of the squat brick houses surrounding the garden, helping me forget that I was, when I moved in, a thirty-three-year-old man living primarily off my father's dwindling inheritance, bound to this city of soot-choked, narrow streets lined in unrelenting rows of red brick, city of dead ends and vacant lots, all like an allegory of my failures to finish either my first book or the academic dissertation I'd meant as the more honorable substitute for that book. Hard to know when exactly I'd fallen into the habit of failure, of leaving everything half done or worse. It used to be that I worked in order to keep up appearances, whether it was my high school biology reports, or the essay on Mallarmé written a week after my father's death. But once my work started to become the purpose itself, once it reflected on me instead of deflecting other people, it began to feel threatening, the stakes too high. Work had been my distraction, but then I began to crave distraction from work, pursuing those distractions with the same intensity and self-absence that used to be part of my working life.

I could forget, too, sometimes for hours, that I was there because I'd followed a woman whose love I'd exhausted. My girlfriend had been offered a coveted tenure-track professorship at the University of Pennsylvania, and her thesis about surviving tragedy was about to be published. We were supposed to have been "queen and king of our own Republic of Letters," as someone had drunkenly said in a toast at our wedding, an alliance of two emotionally fragile creatures. We were stepping hand in hand into the unknown, leaving all the unhappiness and irresolution of our separate childhoods behind us.

Now, in our daughter's darkened bedroom, I lie atop the inherited orientals on the toy-crowded floor, tracing patterns on them in the dark, a not wholly unhappy prisoner of her wishes.

"What do you want to know?" I ask her.

"What did you have for lunch?" she asks.

"What did I have for lunch when I was in kindergarten? It was so long ago," I say. Really, I ought to be briskly kissing her good night and leaving her to learn to tell her own stories in her own space. Instead, nightly, but only three times weekly, for a while longer, I keep her company until she drifts off.

Could she really expect me to remember a lunch eaten nearly thirty years ago, as though I were the same person? But then, as if her question has merely pushed at a door never properly closed, I'm opening a red plastic *The Empire Strikes Back* lunch box by its white clasp, removing a small beige thermos I'm pleased to find my mother has filled with alphabet soup, and a plastic bag containing a salami sandwich with a little bit of butter spread over the wheat bread—the salami smells concentrated in the sealed plastic bag. "Were the crusts cut off?" my daughter wants to know. "I can't remember," I tell her, "but there were usually two small chocolate chip cookies, or something like that." "Is this real?" she asks. I tell her that I can't say for sure that I had this exact lunch on an exact date, and it might have been second grade, because I'm also now remembering the sunflower-yellow shirts with the school's name in dark blue that we wore to gym then—the distinctness of colors in childhood—and Monsieur Valéry, not the poet but our gym teacher, standing in front of the back entrance to the school in his shorts, his soccer-playing thighs bared in even the coldest weather, and hustling us all down the iron fire stairs into the basement, but the lunch box, I tell her, the lunch box was real, and so was the alphabet soup, I'll stand by those. "Did Viki make it for you?" she asked.

"Yes," I say.

"Did she make you lunch every day?"

"Just about," I say.

"Why are you mad at Viki?"

"Oh, sweetheart, it's a long story."

"But she's your mom, you shouldn't be mad at her."

"I'm not mad at her," I lie, "I've just lost patience with her."

"Like you lose patience with me when we're late for school?"

"No, not like that."

"I don't think you should be mad at Viki."

"You may be right, my love, but now it's time to sleep."

"Will you tell me the cloud story?"

As I tell her the cloud story, in which the large and once scary-seeming patch of peeled ceiling plaster above her bed becomes a soft, flying-carpet cloud, taking her off to anodyne thoughts, pastoral landscapes of poppies and grazing unicorns by a mountainside temple, a sound of distant surf lapping in her ears, in which nothing takes place but the place, no harm or action in this spell, while I listen for the sound of her breathing going soft and slow and regular into sleep, I'm also carried off or back by her questions, her uncanny humane intuitions, musing on her insistence on proper names, not "Grandmother," but Viki, just as she's recently insisted on calling me Marco, "Daddy" only to her friends. She seems to have grasped so quickly what it has taken me years to discover: that we are fundamentally separate individuals, not just mere sets of relations. Yet this distinctness is something we perceive only in intimacy, at the same time as our growing intimacy clouds our perceptions of the person's independent qualities. The people we love get reduced to functions and become invisible as individuals—daughter, daddy, mommy, wife, now ex-wife, now only her mother.

Perhaps such advanced knowledge of fragile human individuality is what people mean when they speak about the awful, threatened knowingness of children of divorce. Already she's

seen one unit of stable meaning dissolve, the same actors reap-
pearing on her life's scene, just not in exactly the same roles, and
so already she reaches behind our family masks toward the ultimate mask, what the grandfather she'll never know called "the
person." And so, too, behind her need to know why I'm mad at
Viki, I hear an echo of fear, whether mine or hers it's hard to say:
if I've fallen out so thoroughly with these women in our life, her
mother, her grandmother, what keeps the same fate from befall-
ing her? It's not a question I have an easy answer for. I'm primed
to expect, despite my countless promises not to do unto as was
done, that I will commit only a variant evil. It's not as though
I've never met a father capable of disowning his child, or at least
threatening to do so.

I fear appearing to her just as my father had wanted to appear to me, fixed in an unending hypocrisy: fatherhood as a social category, timeless, stable, unauthored, the father as such,
until he was no longer able to and the masked slipped, when the
vengeful and disappointed man behind the father rose up in him,
as it might in me, too, at any moment of weakness.

To my continual amazement, my child relieves me of that
fear. Instead of condemning me to a perpetual present of "let's
pretend" fatherhood, she's allowed me to link myself with the
child who carried a red lunch box to school. And out of the child
who emerges from her questions comes a fuller truth about myself and about my parents than I was perhaps ready to acknowledge. I don't mean to suggest that I'm redeemed by some sort of
weak inner-childism, that there's still hope for me, too, because
my mother once packed me lunch. But, by putting me back in
touch with that child I once was, my child permits me to share a
life with her in which I can take the proper measure of what was
actually lost. In such moments, I'm released from the feeling that
I've been condemned to rewrite, automatically and unwillingly,
those losses, those accidents and events, real and imagined, into
everything I do, every relationship, every situation, to generalize

my first impressions of emptiness and betrayal and fill the world with the images of those disappointments and my failures to overcome them, again and again.

Also, by this point, I not only believe I know what was lost but what our family never had. I lost patience with my mother because she finally made me a present of the truth, a truth learned too late for my incomplete book about my father's books, and my marriage, and also too late for the happily lonely family of 88 Central Park West. It was as though I simply leaned one day against a familiar wall, expecting its usual weight of resistance, only to have it give way under the merest ordinary pressure, and lead me, stumbling, face-planting, onto the floor of another once-invisible, junk-filled room. Before I could say whether I'd been injured, all I saw were old dust motes stirring, visible suddenly in the unexpected sunlight, swirling into a series of repeating patterns.

My father had been dead thirteen years; my aunt had written four more books in the seven years since her memoir was published. It was a year and a half since my wife had given birth to our daughter, over my worries and objections, and four years since I'd consigned my notes in the brown folder to the same trunk I'd once taken with me to college and had trundled everywhere since, its contents swelling with the weight of the imperfectly executed fodder of my disappointments.

I was up in New York on one of those deceptive warm days in late January, ostensibly to help out with the magazine I'd started with a friend from graduate school and three of his friends from college. We weren't sure if it would last or become a mere gesture of the anger and frustration we'd been carrying around: our disgust at what America was becoming, at what the culture we'd worked to achieve our place in was becoming: the wars, the inequality, the torture and legitimized cruelty, and our own inability to do anything but pursue the narrow careerism of our fragile individual lives, to censor ourselves and obey the rules. The magazine, for the first time, gave me a way to channel my demons of negativity into critique instead of self-destruction.

Its survival beyond the first issue had surprised me and had more to do with my colleagues, each of whom was as used to making things work as I was to undermining myself. As the train rolled out of the industrial ruins of North Philadelphia, I couldn't help feeling they wouldn't have minded if I remained a remote and shadowy contributor, leaving the office to them, but I really needed a break from my marriage. My wife and I were abandoning each other by accusing each other of abandonment, and it seemed wisest, at that point, to take an actual step away.

With my usual ambivalence, I'd accepted my mother's invitation to stay. She said she was planning to cook dinner for us. I arrived early and saw that the table was already elaborately set for two, with an open bottle of wine breathing in the center. I poured myself a glass, walked into the kitchen, and startled my mother where she sat, her small frame buried between stacks of *The New York Times* and mixed old *New Yorker* and *Scientific American* magazines, at a low kidney-shaped table grafted to the kitchen wall of her new apartment. It was the only place to sit there, but placed in a way that left you staring at the blank wall and the row of cabinets over your head. These were all about six feet off the ground and my mother stood little over five feet. In the ten years she'd lived there, she would often say she was planning to redo the kitchen. She also occasionally said she wanted to tear down a wall that separated the living room from the corner room she used to store the extra furniture from our old apartment and inherited from her parents.

She jumped when I greeted her, as if I were a ghost, as if we both knew that I shouldn't have been there at all. She was in the middle of writing a condolence note for Anne's husband, my uncle. He'd been surprised by a heart attack on his way home from a concert with my aunt. A vigorous eighty-one at the time, he'd walked daily to his office, where, until the last day of his life, he psychoanalyzed the children of New York City.

Her stationery was laid out with what I assumed to be a certain grim satisfaction. This was to be her first communication with my aunt, both of them equally widowed now, since the publication of *1185 Park Avenue*. Despite living three blocks from each other, they managed never to cross paths. This was an incredible feat for New York, which, despite the cliché about the city of eight million anonymous faces, is a city of hundreds of villages that generate the unexpected "run-in" with alarming frequency. In my mother's neighborhood, everyone went to the same French bakery, the same supermarket, the same subway and bus stops, the same paths down to the park on the same rare beautiful days. Given the regularity with which my mother ran into these people, I couldn't understand how she and my aunt had managed their feat of avoidance. But after waiting all this time, my mother could at last speak her mind and take some kind of revenge. On the other hand, it was possible that my uncle's death had once more humanized my aunt in my mother's eyes.

I asked what she'd written. She held out the note, and I skimmed it for signs showing that she was really better than my aunt after all, that she'd kept her dignity by remaining silent until she had something important to say, ready to forgive her because they were both sufferers. The letter recalled the recipes she and my uncle had exchanged, the baseball games he'd taken me to without mentioning the incident at the Yankees game that had embarrassed my father. That was it. A man's life becomes cranberry bread and a pitying kindness to a seven-year-old boy raised in a way he disapproved of. It wasn't that the letter felt inevitably formulaic and dry, but somehow it was off-key, without sympathy for either my aunt or my cousins. Oddly like a thank-you letter.

After my father's death, my mother and I had become self-styled connoisseurs of the condolence note. As they'd come in, we'd scrutinized them for signs of the writer's motives. "I'm sorry to hear about your loss . . ." meant that the writer wasn't sorry for the death but for getting news of it; he'd been shaken out of his ordinary complacency and wrote almost as though warding off the evil eye. Most of the notes we got began with expressions of shock. This hadn't been surprising, since there were fewer than ten people who'd known about my father's illness. There were old friends who were hurt to realize that they were out of the loop, that it was now too late to get back in, and they told us so, as if my father's death had wronged them.

Our favorite genre of condolence note was the one that recalled some detail of my father's life, an anecdote from his medical student days or his college years, or recorded my father's kind acts, hidden from us: his care of a particular patient, his vigorous promotion of his former lab technician who'd gone on to become a successful researcher herself.

I recognized my mother's note as intended in this last style. Even so, that genre no longer seemed appropriate. My mother would have been entitled to write "Now you know how it feels!" which wouldn't have been nice, but it would have forced her to acknowledge that Anne was susceptible to feelings. Instead, she bypassed her altogether. She wrote to celebrate and mourn the dead man for what he'd meant to her, although in an elliptical way, also assuming what he'd meant to me. In every other case, that would have been enough, a demonstration of tact, but with the history between them something more was required, or nothing at all.

These thoughts all passed through my head in an inarticulate blink. I doubt I could have put them together. "You're still angry at her" was all I managed to say. My mother looked at me, as if she were reminding herself that my uncle's baseball invitation hadn't arrived the previous week, and nodded.

Whatever it was in that look of hers, fear or guilt, something no longer made sense to me: How could one be enduringly angry at someone who did not, in the end, have either right or power on her side? My aunt was a fantasist, a novelist, an embroiderer of reality, and she'd just been confronted with a loss whose reality could not be denied or pushed away. She had no more influence over us from where she was now. The unprovable speculations she'd published about my father were years behind us, and no one seemed to have made anything out of it, or cared much, really, whether my father had got AIDS in the more usual way; as far as I knew, at least, no one cared about it apart from us.

Surely my mother, who appeared to have remained so constant and close to my father that she still hadn't remarried or even so much as dated regularly, my mother, who I knew kept boxes in closets, still unpacked from our first move, several drawers full of my old toys, photographs of my father displayed next to the piano in the living room, of me, too, but none in which I was older than seven—with the recent exception of a soon-to-be-obsolete wedding photo—my mother, who slept on a twin-sized daybed in a room intended to be the study, dominated by floor-to-ceiling bookshelves packed mostly with my father's books, which she neither read nor threw away—surely she must have found some strength in this great enduring love for the man she'd married. At that moment, however, something made me turn back. I asked again the same question I'd asked in the dosa restaurant, years before, or rather I asked it in a different, more direct way: "Were you telling me the truth?"

Instead of answering, my mother asked if I wanted to go for a walk—which was her way of saying that she wanted to go for a walk. I was reminded of one of my father's apparently endless supply of jokes, of which I'd retained so few: The Russian ambassador to Washington calls his wife in Moscow to see how everything's going. "Grigori," she tells him, "I have bad news: Molotov fell off the roof and died."

Molotov was the ambassador's old cat, and the ambassador gets very upset. "Katia, oh my heart, how many times do I have to tell you never to give me bad news like this. You know about my condition. This is not how you're supposed to deliver it."

"Forgive me, Grigori, what should I have said?"

"Oh, you're an idiot and a good woman. Why didn't you tell me that the cat is on the roof, that he's been up there for a while. The neighbors have been trying to get him to come down, but he's resisting, clawing and spitting, tough old cat that he is. Then say that it started to rain. Maybe he'll come down now. And then, only then, do you tell me that he slipped, and then tell me that he only hurt his paw, that the veterinarian is coming, and then the veterinarian comes, and then you say, like it was nothing, that you buried him yesterday under the cherry tree by the dacha. Finished. That's how you do it, Katia darling. But let's talk about something else. How is our dear Comrade Brezhnev?"

"Grigori, Comrade Brezhnev is on the roof."

We went out, flashing faux cheer at Eduardo, the doorman, as he called out "Ms. Viki, Mr. Marco, so good to see you." I wondered what he could see that made us seem so happy. Over the years, my mother and I have grown to look increasingly like brother and sister. Her unruly curls are dyed a subtle shade of auburn. There's as much gray in them as in my own, or less. She walks lightly and quickly. Yoga and the Alexander Technique taught her to hold herself straight and supple with the ease of a thirty-year-old. No surgeon's knife has lifted her face, but I've often thought she looks younger in her sixties than she did in the photographs I've seen of her in her thirties. It's as though she remembered how to smile.

I was bringing all her burdens back to her, unwelcomed. I often thought she'd be better if she cut me off and really started a new life. We were unpleasant and awkward around each other. She was afraid of me, I could tell, and that fear enraged me. She would have preferred an aimless meander down to Riverside Park, a remark on the weather. She would have listened to me talk about her adored granddaughter, then two, the modest success of the magazine, or Beethoven trios. But I kept a deliberate silence. We walked slowly. I smoked in front of her, knowing she'd be upset by it, but hoping it would bring her to the point faster.

We were halfway around the block, down by the promenade above Riverside Park, and I was on my second cigarette before she started, at last. "Dad loved you, loved us," she began, as she'd begun before, and, as before, I cut her off. "That's not what I asked." We walked on in silence, anxiously down past my aunt's apartment building, toward the Fireman's Memorial. We rounded the corner, heading back up to West End Avenue, back toward the apartment and the disquieting silence we'd started out from, silence redoubled. My mother plunged again, she said, "In, I guess, 1976, you were about two, Dad, Gene, your father, told me he'd been . . . sleeping . . . with a man, but that he'd stopped and it was the last time. Maybe he kept his promise, maybe he didn't. Maybe that was the truth, maybe that wasn't the whole truth." She continued, "When you asked me before what I knew about how he got AIDS and I said I knew what you knew, I was telling you the truth."

How does one begin to recall a conversation like this? I wasn't taking notes, and I wasn't listening with an ear for posterity. I was in the middle of it. Disconnected phrases float up, but these memories aren't entirely misleading. My mother seemed unsure what voice to use, whether she should speak as a mother, reassuring the boy I no longer was about a father who had been gone awhile, whose abandonment was accidental and unintended. "Dad loved you, loved us," a mantra, the way the self-help literature recommends that we tell children of divorce that it's not their fault in such a way that can only make them think the opposite. Abruptly, though, within the pauses, she'd shift, as though confiding in a skeptical friend or a psychoanalyst. "I knew when I married him, but I can be very stubborn. When I was three years old, my father's business associate Michael and his friend Herschel often came to visit us. And you know that Michael and Herschel were . . . I guess what we'd now call partners . . . Michael was wonderful to me. So kind. And I, I really loved Michael." And, at last, with a sigh, almost of impatience, "I thought you really always must have known."

Had I been stupid, blundering and insensitive? Up rose a flash of memory showing me my father reading the gay British historian A. L. Rowse's *Homosexuals in History*. It was tented open, the front cover a photo of Michelangelo's David, glorious nudity right there on the bed. Right there an invitation, perhaps, for me to ask why he was reading it. I had filed it under general culture, the library of every civilized person. I had missed everything, missed my parents' lives.

We went back upstairs to the new apartment, which, more than ever, struck me as a condensed version of our former Central Park West one, a miniature museum to a past that seemed to have been nothing but a hoax, our Oblomovka. The dinner things were still out on the table, untouched, shimmering before my eyes. I picked up a half-full glass of wine, twirled it, and hurled it against the wall, uncertain if it would break or, as if in some science fiction movie, keep traveling, sole substantial thing in this illusory world.

Dutifully, but without any real remorse and even a certain feeling of relief (at least that's out of the way!), I swept up the fragments and vacuumed shards and splinters and sponged the wall clean of stain, but, to save my embarrassment, and in the name of artfulness, permit me an extra level of allegory out of this tantrum.

Let's hold up a surprisingly intact piece from the wineglass bowl and look at my mother through it, glued wordlessly to an armchair. She'd obviously just done, for her, an enormously brave thing, one of the bravest in her life. She must have known she was taking a huge risk telling me when she'd told me. Not only disgorging a painful secret, a secret that she'd kept faithfully for years and which had come to keep her in turn, the secret that served as the holy of holies of our otherwise unreligious and ritual-free family life, but she was also admitting her earlier lie. She must have felt as though she were walking barefoot over all those scattered shards. Impossible to say whether she was in fact acknowledging, really, fully, for the first time, that she'd resented my father cheating on her, if we can call it cheating to be with someone who gives you what your wife couldn't possibly, even if she wanted to. Impossible to say, too, when she must have understood that any future relationship with me and with the granddaughter whose infant stubbornness, she said, reminded her of her own, required that she sacrifice this idol of her past.

Only later did I realize that my mother's confession was a surrender of her power to me. Our family happiness or unhappiness was in my hands, depended on my responses. I did not even thank her for coming clean. In the moment, I couldn't have cared what my mother was enduring. In the brittleness of those first minutes, I was insulted she'd failed to trust me, back when my aunt had published her book. My mother tried to persuade me that I shouldn't take it personally. It was the era, she said. Not so much today as the '50s, the long reach of America's conformist decade. Everyone was afraid. That had been my aunt's line, too, about "bending under the deceptions forged in crueler times," as though my parents or rather my family were merely victims of preenlightened conditions. This was also, as far as I was concerned, bullshit historicism. The sociology was another fancy way of making excuses, outsourcing a decision to some higher power. Cowardice is cowardice. "Don't ask, don't tell" was a policy for the military, not the family, and a misguided one. Neither did we live among the kind of people who thought AIDS was God's tough-love epistle to the queers. If the Upper West Side of Manhattan in the 1980s and early 1990s was not a safe enough milieu to discuss homosexuality with one's child, then nowhere was. There had only been me, myself, standing for nothing, representing no one else, no social movement or political party. Change has to begin somewhere, I said to my mother, and if times have changed it's because other people were better than we were.

She admitted it. But there were things, she said, that she still believed no child really ought to know about his or her parents, that were, essentially, none of my business. It was, she repeated, her life. Before my eyes, she was retreating back to where she'd been before, as if once the glass were cleaned up we could simply go on forgetting about it. The bedroom door was closed.

In a way my mother was right . . . if we'd been a normal family . . . if such a thing indeed existed . . . the taboo against talking to your kids too much about who likes what where, with whom, and how is something to be respected. In a world so thoroughly sexualized now, in which we're always being told to enjoy our drives, the family, perversely, might be the last place on earth that offers us the freedom to think about something other than sex.

My mother was also being honorable, like the heroine of a stately, aristocratic tragedy by Racine. Even after our traditional family was no longer traditional, she would not have violated the rule, risked bringing about something new. But I was burned out from her noblesse. I thought of her, at first, as if she were acting like a patient my father used to tell us about when he'd come home from the sickle-cell clinic: Mr. Adams, a recent convert to Islam, had stopped taking his sickle-cell medication because he worried the pills contained pork gelatin. He'd appealed to my father as a Jew—"Jews don't eat the pig neither, Dr. Roth"—and my father had tried to explain that any ethical rabbi would offer a special dispensation to violate dietary laws in cases of life and death. To which Mr. Adams answered, "That's where the imam goes the rabbi one better, he don't care if you die, you just can't eat pork."

My mother had also bettered the rabbi. But if our family could have survived, not just my father's death, but all the events that led up to it, someone needed to have suspended the ordinary rules of reticence and pretense. The great mystery into which I'd at last, bumblingly, been initiated was not just sex or desire or the mysteries of human attraction and attractiveness. Among all the smithereens, I understood I'd broken through, at last, to the essence of the thwartedness that clung to my parents' lives, to my life with my parents. This, I suppose, was what I'd always known, even if I hadn't known that I knew it. I remembered a former writing instructor's impatient comments on the early stories I'd written for "Structure and Style": "Nothing happens!"; "Pay attention to plot, motive, action!"; "Scenes are about people wanting things!" For me, home had been the place where nothing happened and to want was straightaway to be disappointed.

It occurred to me, too, that this feeling of nothing happening was exactly how my parents had wanted it. Both of them. They were kept safe from what they most desired and most feared, and this contagion of safety, of enclosure, they'd communicated to me, insidiously, without any of us having a choice in the matter. I'd been right to think that they'd deliberately prepared me for a future of disappointment, of a museumlike world of cultural and other goods that I'd never be able to touch or really experience or make for myself. I was wrong that they'd done it deliberately. The taboo under which they both lived had become a generalized "Thou shalt not want," overshadowing everything to which I put my hand.

My mother rose up from the chair, went into the kitchen, and came back holding open a garbage bag for me to dump in the swept-up shards. I thanked her.

"Why do you have to get so angry like that?" she asked. It was the first time she'd asked.

"I'm sorry . . ." I said, "about the glass."

"Your great-grandmother . . ."

"I know." I stroked my mother's hair the way I stroked the hair of my child as she was going to sleep.

13

That night, in the bed that had been my childhood bed and my mother's before that, I recalled something like a paranormal event, a dream I'd had a few weeks after my father's death. I'd been back at 88 Central Park West for some reason, packing maybe, and I'd gone into the music room to do some course reading and lain down on the same black leather couch where I'd waited while my father had prepared his final medication. It was an afternoon near the winter solstice, but in that room, with its six large windows facing Central Park, there was always enough natural light to read. Still, I couldn't follow the book, my thoughts wandered, I closed my eyes. Several weeks dead, my father walked into the room: "You need more light," he said. I woke up; the sun had gone down, and, somehow, the halogen floor lamp by the room's arched entryway, a good ten feet from the couch, had been turned up all the way.

Whatever the explanation—sleepwalking, the light had been on the whole time and I noticed it only once it was dark, my mother had come in while I was already asleep, thinking I was still reading—I certainly had more light now. It was only a matter of learning how or what to read by it. Inevitably the thought came that I had to set the story down in some way: not with any particular agenda as in some La Fontaine animal fable to show that "Secrets Are Wrong," or "Outmoded Taboos and Prejudices

About Homosexuality Destroy Lives!" Or: "Parents! Do Not Lie
to Your Children, Ever!" And not, at last, to get back at anyone,
least of all my mother for lying, for I, too, was to blame for the
days that had become months that had become years of sitting
in rooms, turning the pages in search of an answer that might
have come to me sooner if I'd somehow been able to convince
my parents of my trustworthiness.

Or maybe my fault was the opposite: that I respected them
too much to want to make them an object of my own private
inquiry and exposé, and yet didn't really respect them enough to
have secured myself a truly happy false memory of my childhood that proofed me against any future revelations. In the end,
I'd gone about things lazily and sneakily, as I'd snuck my way
into Columbia and taken my father's money without wanting to
give up either my sense of autonomy or my belief that I was a
victim of circumstances. How easy it turns out to be to want
things both ways! If I wanted to be kinder to myself, I could say
that I'd done things indirectly, the long way, which is almost the
wrong way but not quite.

Inevitably the thought also came to me that I mustn't write
about any of this. That such an act was what my parents most
dreaded. My mother was doubly doomed to live it again, and so
was I, unless . . . Unless I went my own way with an equal violence, which I seemed unable to do, and which seemed somehow
anyway impossible. After all, I had to live with this knowledge,
too, as my mother had lived with it. On top of that, I felt the
weight of all my wasted time: those months and years of my fur-
tive reading, the truncated writing, the head-banging frustration
of not getting anywhere and not getting away.

Perhaps, too, their arrangement had suited them. Perhaps if
there'd been no HIV, my father would have gone on, more or less
happily, in his double life, flown off to Morocco for some interna-
tional hematology conference and brought back a pair of camel-
hide slippers for me, an inlaid silver bracelet for my mother, and

his own memories. Or he might have come out of the closet, eventually, when I was teenager, moved in with a young Asian violinist a little older than I was, and I would have become ferociously jealous, joined a college fraternity, gone off on some confused, gay-bashing prank with all my new brothers, and ended up embittered in a totally different way. There were myriad possible variations but only one real outcome. I'd been the child of their denial. I knew that now. I could become, in a way, and perhaps for the first time, no longer a guest in my parents' house.

But in what ways were most of us not the children of denial? That's what civilization was supposed to be. We didn't run around getting whatever we wanted whenever we wanted it. The feeling that sexual preferences cannot be sacrificed was new to the later twentieth century, but it was not always a moral wrong to sacrifice a shot at wild ecstasy for the sake of the philosophic mind. What I found so shocking, so enraging about my parents was that they appeared to have had no conscious awareness of the moral dimension of their decisions. My mother had invested so much in getting me to believe we were all leading exactly the life we wanted without compromise and disappointment, and this was so obviously untrue that I had no idea what to make of it.

I awoke the next morning thinking everything had changed. And yet nothing changes right away, at least not dramatically. I padded carefully through the living room in case of any stray glass splinters, greeted my mother in her office behind the kitchen where she was already e-mailing various contacts, trying to get them to sponsor a contemporary composer. She told me she'd made coffee, although if she hadn't I would have thought something was really amazingly amiss. I walked out and took the subway to the magazine's Lower East Side office, where I intended to revise an essay I was writing about why clones had started appearing in self-consciously literary fiction.

Swaying to the familiar rhythms of the D train, I looked at my fellow morning riders with more than my habitual, half-lustful eye. Since my father's death and the waning of the AIDS plague in the well-heeled capitals of world finance, it was as if a whole host of unwritten sumptuary laws had been handed down, replacing older restrictions with the far more difficult command that everyone should dress in ways that were supposed to make them feel good about themselves and make everyone feel good about everyone else. There was no one in the subway car like my father, with his slightly baggy suits, his mismatched ties, slouching or hunching into and away from his body.

In the false spring weather, most of the passengers were turned out for New York's magical moment of sexual utopianism. Bespoke suits radiated imperturbable mastery alongside skirts in lengths and materials from demure to dominatrix; slim-cut oxfords and tight muscle tees rubbed against backless dresses and plunging halter tops as pairs of tight jeans, bulged at the crotch or the ass, letting slip a ribbon of tattooed skin, sought warmth against fuzzy polar fleeces and pole-danced in the middle of the car next to thrift-store and vintage specials. Everything seemed to fit too tightly.

As New York subways often do, the train lurched to a stop in the middle of a tunnel. The passengers in their sudden helplessness began to eye one another a bit more openly, unsure whether it was some disaster or attack we were all dimly anticipating or the more ordinary red signal. In the stilled motion of the car, I began to drift off. From the doors connecting the cars, I conjured a crack team of shrinks—not the celebrity Dr. Phils, or the pillmongers, and not my old Freudian Dr. Z with his Oedipal remedies, but a cast of Lacanians, Kleinians, and Winnicotians devoted to consciousness as an ongoing process of self-discovery rather than some idea of "mental health." They waded into the crowd, waving their notebooks, organizing the passengers into some new, Delphic rite of self-knowledge. "Tell us your fantasies for love and work," they'd say, "or tell us your fears, share something of your core self. If you want to crawl on the floor and

scream like a baby, that's fine. Whatever takes you at this moment. If you want to switch clothes with your neighbor, ask her
or him. No murders allowed, and, please, any consensual sexual
encounters should take place when the séance is over, even if you
happen to be exhibitionists, and even though we doubt any of
you can really consent consciously to anything. That's why we're
here and that's why you're all here, trapped in this car. Whatever
it is you do at this moment will reveal something about yourself
you were unaware of. This train to nowhere will change your life."

What would I do as the shrinks approached me? I thought
for a moment, and realized I really just wanted to argue with
them. "Come on, these are my fantasies. But I like my fantasies
because they're my fantasies. What happens once I expose them
under the bright white lights and advertisements of this car?
They'll become subject to the same fearful and boring realities
I've designed these fantasies to escape from. What about them?"
I would say, catching sight of a young man I hadn't noticed before, sitting slouched with tie askew, jacket folded over one arm,
pressed uncomfortably against a taller woman who wore a tight
1960s miniskirt, her long bare legs pressed together, an unlit
cigarette dangling from her lips, her hair in a dark bob that hid
its natural waves. They whispered to each other, and he said something that made her laugh: my father and my aunt, as they were
in their twenties. "Do you think that anything other than time
will show this woman, who thinks of herself as a novelist, that
she's really a scientist, fueled by doubts and determined to find
truths, no matter how uncomfortable? Or that her brother, next
to her, might really be a most remarkable kind of artist, for whom
the study of actual cell biologies, studies to which he'll devote
years of his life, is only a single part of an elaborate performance,
a performance so successful that he'll manage to convince many
that it's a life more real and certainly less hypocritical than many,
and yet a life given also to the creation and maintenance of what
turns out to have been a counterlife, a caretaker life that protects

him against what he knows he wants, while also protecting those same wants, allowing them to remain intact as desires and fantasies, living on within him until they burst out with a force that will mar at least three lives . . ."

Like adult forms of the HIV virus from the immune cells whose DNA helped create them, I thought, as the train jerked back into its regular rhythm. The crowd of shrinks vanished. My father and my aunt were nowhere to be found. I reminded myself to be careful with those cellular similes. AIDS was no more a punishment hatched in my father's id or handed down from the pagan fates of narrative justice than it ever was "God's punishment." Making the random mutation of a microscopic virus into the retrospective master text was a constant temptation and the last taboo. And yet that's what people do: we can't not want there to be metaphors, even as we know there's a gap between metaphor and reality that can trip us up, like the gap between train and station platform that I stepped over without even noticing as I sprang up the steps out of the Second Avenue station, exiting by the busy playground and handball courts that stretched along the north side of Houston Street, formerly a gathering spot for junkies and dealers. It was here, or not far from here, I imagined, in the mid-1980s, that my aunt's oldest daughter had shared a needle or met a man who shared a needle, a scant few blocks from where our common ancestor had plied his pushcart.

Whether it was because she was younger, her HIV diagnosed earlier, her will to live stronger, or the strain of the virus weaker, my cousin survived long enough for scientists to figure out more precise and potent combinations of reverse transcriptase inhibitors and other drugs. The cocktail, as it came to be known, was not a single dramatic cure, but it allowed her and others to live on, a trace amount of the virus remaining inside them, almost, but never exactly, tamed.

As I could not have known when I wrote my teenage report, I saw that there had always been hope, only not for many of us.

Even in this cleaned-up aftermath, where kids raced over the syringe-free asphalt, in this supposedly happiest of countries, where freedom, democracy had triumphed over communism, that mutant strain of freedom and democracy, where scientists worked daily to crack the codes of all our microscopic enemies, no one had managed to cure us of the desire for the shared needle, or the wrong man at the wrong time, the inappropriate association.

If I was going to delve deeply into my father's fate, I could not just assume, as my aunt had assumed, that he was merely chained by the memory of a childhood shame of his exposed love for other boys, the victim of cultural prejudices about homosexuals, driven to seek furtively and unsafely what he now could have had for the asking: the right to love after his own fashion. No, I had to consider that he'd been afraid of something really worth being afraid of, and that his fear led him into marriage, into fatherhood, into his lab among the mice, mosquitoes, and parasites he cultivated and destroyed with such admirable, dispassionate intensity, so that the obstacles between himself and his desire were multiplied like the concentric walls of a dungeon from which he nevertheless managed to escape into what was only another dungeon, deeper down.

My aunt had taught me that I could not shirk a duty to my own worst thoughts, that I must, as she would say, consider the possibility that whatever my father sought, wherever he sought it, he wanted to be mortified, hurt. Somewhere in him, before the disease, was a craving to suffer that no mere change in social attitudes or emancipatory laws could take away. This was what no one had wanted to think about, because it was almost unthinkable.

Of course I could have decided to go looking for some more concrete proof, although the odds of finding anything definitive seemed very poor. I could no longer talk to Victor, who'd succumbed to early-onset Alzheimers. I pictured myself walking around New York like a private investigator carrying a picture of my father from the 1970s—"Have you seen this man?"—tracking down former frequenters of "Cell Block 28," the Ansonia bath-house, five blocks from our old apartment, or the uptown down-low clubs closer to the sickle-cell clinic where my father had worked, except that these clubs, too, were gone, along with most of the people who'd frequented them, including whoever had passed the disease on to my father.

I'd reached an area of darkness in which the more I learned, the less I could say that I really knew. It was the closest I'd come to something like the full truth. Fortunately, I'd also reached the magazine's office. A sublet room on an airshaft in a warrenlike building that mixed together illegal-immigrant-staffed sweat-shops, metalworkers, small publishers, musicians, modeling agen-cies that may or may not have been porn-industry fronts, and squatters who occupied several of the unrented studios. It was still early in the morning, by our standards; our business man-ager and my fellow editors didn't usually show up before eleven o'clock, although I half expected to find one of them asleep on the couch after an all-nighter of proofreading. I started over to the computer to begin entering changes to my piece, but my attention was caught by a pile of thick envelopes, unopened and stacked by the door. I began to open them, mechanically. Mostly these were books that publishers had begun sending to us, unsolicited, for review.

There were so many of them, and more on our shelves, and more arriving each day, which was strange, since we'd begun the magazine in what was considered a period of crisis for literature. We were living in the age of "the death of the book," we kept hearing, or, worse "the end of reading." Panels were convened, essays commissioned, surveys released. The terminal mood was inescapable. And yet there were still so many books. I supposed one could see them as the hyperventilating of a dying patient, gasping for more breath, clinging tenaciously to the moments before the final tracheal rattle, or like a last glorious hemorrhage of voices, stained bright, frothing out before a final silence. But an idea, or a form, or a way of life does not dramatically expire. It persists as itself and not itself, like the looming shadow of the hidden water tower that once made me think I was going blind.

When people spoke of the death of the book, they really seemed to be mourning the loss of a set of fantasies about literature. The realization that books were a mere technology, something between a widget and an automobile, susceptible to obsolescence, was like the last thunk of earth, a recognition that the promises of the literary liberal culture of my father and aunt's generation had not been kept, perhaps could never have been kept, and, in fact, had been made to be broken. Reading was not automatically going to make you a better person, it was not an ineluctable path to self-knowledge; if it could make you sympathetic to other people, that sympathy was still unlikely to translate into meaningful solidarity and political action; it was not going to make you more successful at your job or happier in your sex life.

It occurred to me that I'd been stalling my own reckoning with the future of literature by transplanting literature into my father's life. I'd been using him, in a way, or using his memory. Not maliciously, but in order to keep alive a flickering sense of connection to a history that had really been neither mine nor my father's but had become our only shared connection after hope of all other connection was lost. In the same way, too, he'd used me—*"La Cigale ayant chanté / Tout l'été"*—so I wouldn't be just his son but also La Fontaine's and Thomas Mann's and Goncharov's and Proust's. Things had got now to the point where I could no more disassociate these books from my own fate than I could detach them from my father's.

Over the years since I'd last stood at my father's grave, meditating on his redemption and my eventual emancipation from my family's web of influences, hints, and unstated duties, I'd thought of the book I was going to write as the end of my un- accomplished mourning, the unsaid Kaddish that could not, even later, be said, the resumption of the burial once left to more hardened hands. That book, too, it became clear to me, would have been only another false memorial to my father's wholly unreconciled life, a pseudo-substitution of culture for a desire that, in the end, accepted no substitutes.

Alone, then, in the few minutes or hours before my friends arrived and the everyday, workaday world started up again, I stretched out in the shadowy and cluttered office room. I began to clear some space, putting the new books on the swelling shelves, wiping the coffee rings and beer rings off our common table. I opened the airshaft window and let in a warm laundry smell and the shouts of Chinese workers from below. Nothing changes right away, least of all a habit of understanding. No, the only thing I could do was go back, once again, retranscribe as much of the whole thing as possible, with an eye for the differ- ence between what we wanted and what we were: a different kind of reverse transcription that allowed me to live detached from what my family had been, what my culture had been, while they still lived on in me, now part of the inalienable matter of my existence. The time was coming closer when I might, at last, put it down.

ACKNOWLEDGMENTS

The author thanks for emotional, intellectual, editorial, and material indulgence and sustenance over the years: Nina Dudás, Imogen Roth, Benjamin Kunkel, Keith Gessen, Nasser Zakariya, Ilya Kliger, Susan Levine, Carol Yaple, Duncan Chesney, Steven Bourke, Ruth Halikman, Emily Wilson, Katie Roiphe, Emily Carter, Andrew Glassman, David Bromwich, Peter Brooks, Idit Alphandary, Sylvère Lotringer, Gayatri Spivak, Joe Schwartz, Stephen Fischer, Craig Arnold, Lorin Stein, Mark Krotov, Marion Duvert, Amy Rosenberg, Siddhartha Deb, Moira Weigel, Sarah Rainone, Jenny Davidson, Maya Jasanoff, Emily Gould, Thomas DeMonchaux, Caleb Crain, Guy Walter, Francine Prose, the Yale Comparative Literature Department, the Pew Center for Arts and Heritage, the editors and staff of *n+1* magazine, Elyse Cheney, Jonathan Galassi, and Victoria Roth.